Praise for
EXPLOITING MY BABY

"Exploiting her baby, perhaps, but most certainly rewarding her readers, Teresa Strasser trudges, nay, romps with us down the road from the anxiety of no baby to guilt of not deserving a precious child. All the while she reminds us that the echoes of our families of origin, although carried along with us like so much muck in a riverbed, need not choke our ability to flourish and find joy as parents." —Dr. Drew Pinsky

"If Woody Allen was a woman with big giant ovaries and wrote a book about his pregnancy, it still wouldn't have been this funny, warm, brassy, and insightful."

—Stefanie Wilder-Taylor, bestselling author of
Sippy Cups Are Not for Chardonnay

"If this is what it's really like to have a baby, I should have been a lot nicer to my lovely wife. Also, she should have made me laugh this much. So we're even. . . . .If you think you worry too much about being a parent, Teresa Strasser will inform you of all the things you forgot to freak out about."

—Joel Stein

"I loved this book. Teresa Strasser has blessed us all with an amazing, inspired work. I laughed, I cried, I learned lessons about marriage and love and pregnancy and motherhood that will last a lifetime. Teresa knows how to speak directly to every one of us, and offers us the inside story every pregnant woman wishes someone out there would finally share. Her very personal, hysterical, and moving story is universal. I can't wait to buy this book for all my pregnant friends."

—Rabbi Naomi Levy, author of *Hope Will Find You* and
To Begin Again

"Teresa is the mom you want to invite to your playgroup."

—Heather McDonald, *New York Times* bestselling author of
You'll Never Blueball in This Town Again

EXPLOITING MY BABY

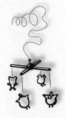

A Memoir of Pregnancy & Childbirth

TERESA STRASSER

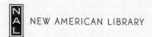
NEW AMERICAN LIBRARY

New American Library
Published by New American Library, a division of
Penguin Group (USA) Inc., 375 Hudson Street,
New York, New York 10014, USA
Penguin Group (Canada), 90 Eglinton Avenue East, Suite 700, Toronto,
Ontario M4P 2Y3, Canada (a division of Pearson Penguin Canada Inc.)
Penguin Books Ltd., 80 Strand, London WC2R 0RL, England
Penguin Ireland, 25 St. Stephen's Green, Dublin 2,
Ireland (a division of Penguin Books Ltd.)
Penguin Group (Australia), 250 Camberwell Road, Camberwell, Victoria 3124,
Australia (a division of Pearson Australia Group Pty. Ltd.)
Penguin Books India Pvt. Ltd., 11 Community Centre, Panchsheel Park,
New Delhi - 110 017, India
Penguin Group (NZ), 67 Apollo Drive, Rosedale, North Shore 0632,
New Zealand (a division of Pearson New Zealand Ltd.)
Penguin Books (South Africa) (Pty.) Ltd., 24 Sturdee Avenue,
Rosebank, Johannesburg 2196, South Africa

Penguin Books Ltd., Registered Offices:
80 Strand, London WC2R 0RL, England

First published by New American Library,
a division of Penguin Group (USA) Inc.

First Printing, January 2011
10 9 8 7 6 5 4 3 2

Copyright © Teresa Strasser, 2011
All rights reserved

 REGISTERED TRADEMARK—MARCA REGISTRADA

LIBRARY OF CONGRESS CATALOGING-IN-PUBLICATION DATA:
Strasser, Teresa.
Exploiting my baby: because it's exploiting me: a memoir of pregnancy & childbirth/Teresa Strasser.
p.   cm.
ISBN 978-0-451-23207-6
1. Mothers—Biography.   2. Motherhood.   3. Pregnancy.   4. Childbirth.   I. Title.
HQ759.S8137 2011
306.874'3092—dc22   2010030897
[B]

Set in Adobe Jenson Pro
Designed by Ginger Legato

Printed in the United States of America

PUBLISHER'S NOTE
Penguin is committed to publishing works of quality and integrity. In that spirit, we are proud to offer this book to our readers; however the story, the experiences and the words are the author's alone.

The publisher does not have any control over and does not assume any responsibility for author or third-party Web sites or their content.

For my husband and baby.
Thanks for letting me exploit you.

CONTENTS

CONTENTS

CONTENTS

About This Book

Why Exploiting My Baby
Seems Like a Good Idea

Like it's so special having a baby. Britney Spears did it twice, so there you go.

Yet we've all seen these spooky, obsessed smother mothers with their sippy cups full of self-absorption and their nonstop, mind-numbing prattle about the relative merits of different brands of organic baby food. These are the souls who update their Facebook status to reflect little Jackson's latest bowel movement. This is not okay. This is chilling.

There are so many nerve-racking things about being pregnant for the first time. Just when you think you can handle nausea, ravenous hunger, precipitous weight gain, and of course the abject fear about your baby's health, you come into contact with one of these mothers and you think, "Not that I'm so great, but I hope I don't become *her.*"

Frankly, before I got pregnant, I was never actually all that comfortable being me, but it was all I knew. Would I now become an uptight asshole who would insist you douse yourself in Purell before touching my offspring, lest you pass on some grubby infection to my precious baby Jesus child? Would I find myself driving a minivan to Tot Shabbat—glassy-eyed and resentful—wearing a crumb-covered Ann Taylor knit and blasting Raffi?

Would all of my concerns in life revolve around what kind of crib mattress was optimum or how best to pack a diaper bag so I could spend the day pushing a stroller through an indoor mall like the other zombie moms, stopping only occasionally to bust out some watermelon cubes from a worn Tupperware container? Would I get gory stretch marks and an eighteen-year-long case of postpartum depression like my mother? Would I feel suffocated and fake a seizure just for some "alone time"?

While I hemorrhaged money on Baby Einstein mobiles and brain-enhancing music classes for the little one, would my own mind atrophy?

In essence: Would both my ass and my mind wear mom jeans?

I had no idea about any of this.

Maybe everything had already been said about the experience of pregnancy, but it was new to me and I found myself not only wanting to write about it but also consuming any information I could, from Nancy O'Dell's book (beautiful lady, but her memoir about extra-glowing pregnancy skin and lack of any unpleasant symptoms can *suck it*) to Jenny McCarthy (you want to dismiss her but you can't, because Jenny is charming and likeable and has touched Oprah with her own hands. Still, her style makes you want to say, "I get it. You're edgy. Even though you're hot, you talk about poops and farts. Goooooood for you").

I sought out books and blogs that would level with me, and I don't mean syrupy pseudo-disclosures like, "I haven't washed my hair in weeks, but it's all worth it because of the majesty of motherhood." I wanted precise details about both the trip and the destination. What *exactly* was going to happen to my digestive system, cervix, weight, delicate internal anxiety management system, boobs, mind, sex life, sense of personal freedom, bladder, marriage, anus, appetite, mood, body image, overall ability to accept changing identity, deeply rooted and unrelenting mommy issues, chronic insomnia, beloved but moderate use of toxins, oil glands, abdomen, shoe size? Who was I going to be on the other side, and how painful would it be crossing over?

As long as there are pregnant girls up in the middle of the night wondering if it's a cramp or gas or a disaster, as long as there are newcomers to this world as confused and terrified as I was, this pregnancy thing is always going to be fresh and relevant.

There is no precedent for us first-timers. I didn't understand any of the sensations happening in my body, which all seemed like they must mean imminent miscarriage, a phrase I Googled no fewer than 137 times.

I didn't have any idea what nipple salve or nasal aspirators do. I didn't know what a doula was, except maybe something you might find on a platter of Mediterranean food. I didn't know anything about babies, except that I was having one. Moreover, I didn't know how to write about any of this without conjuring images of poor, kicked-around Kathie Lee Gifford, who seems like an all right gal but who took so much shit for trotting out little Cody and little what's-her-face just to make America love her.

I guess it seemed like she was just *exploiting* her babies.

Maybe she was, and maybe it was obnoxious for Kathie Lee to use her children to present a sweet, homey version of herself no one was buying. Maybe she truly was a baby-exploiting phony who deserved all the vitriol she got. But when I thought about it, I wasn't totally innocent of my own brand of creative exploitation.

As a writer, I guess I've "exploited" all of my subjects: my stepparents, my boyfriends, my beat-up cars, my jacked-up apartments, my land-lords, my Hebrew school teachers, my grandfather, my girlfriends, the dude at the dry cleaner's, my therapist(s), my dermatologist, the hot guy I met at that silent Buddhist retreat in San Diego, everyone. From breakups to breakdowns, I've always just written about whatever was going on in my life, but because this was a fetus, it suddenly seemed tacky, Kathie Lee tacky.

Sometimes, when you're scared about how something is going to be perceived, you have to look the bogeyman right in the face, which is why at two months pregnant I invested $10 and bought the domain name ExploitingMyBaby.com.

And after all, the kid *was* exploiting me. One day, I thought, "Kid, I just made you a spleen and some eyebrows. The least you can do is get mommy a book deal."

Out in the world of mom-to-be books, I found a gaping hole, a no-man's-land between treacly tales that would make unicorns yak and clinical descriptions of symptoms that are useful, but about as emotionally satisfying as a dental supplies catalogue. I also found a trove of bitter "motherhood sucks" volumes that depressed me when I needed to be feeling okay about the biggest "no *backsies*" decision of my life.

My goal was to trudge the road from conception to delivery, taking good notes as I went and hopefully sharing insights beyond "I pooped on the delivery table." Although, I do have a poop story that I hope will be the number-one story you will ever hear about number two.

These notes and blog posts turned into kind of a memoir, which I hope starts a fruitful lifetime of exploitation. On a less glib front, if you are reading this, you are probably pregnant or planning to be, and I hope I can be a gestational companion. I desperately needed preg-nant friends, and I hope to be one of yours, or at least give you something to do at night when you can't sleep and are sick of reading what food item your fetus most resembles (Your baby is now the size of a poppy seed! A blueberry! A prune! A kiwi! An avocado! A grapefruit! An eggplant! A squash! A watermelon!).

The more I posted, the more women responded, the more I realized I wasn't alone in my neuroses. I knew I was doing the right thing.

So, let the exploitation begin.

EXPLOITING
MY
BABY

Introduction

How No Baby Meant No Job
on *The View*

On New Year's Eve, my husband, Daniel, and I stayed home, ordered Thai food and watched a documentary on Dr. Paul Joseph Goebbels, the minister of propaganda in Nazi Germany. I guess you could say we partied like it was 1939. By my calculations, that's when our baby was conceived.

I immediately started worrying about everything from birth defects to vaginal tearing. I agonized about my lack of ability to make decisions about birth plans, stroller brands or preschools. I had nightmarish visions of morphing into my own cold, reluctant and baby-disdaining mother. About the only thing I didn't worry much about was the prospect of being a working mother in show business. For that, I thank Barbara Walters.

In fact, a few years ago, *not* having a kid may have actually cost me my dream job, filling the chair left by Lisa Ling on *The View*.

I sat in for a couple of episodes, had some wholesome, well-lit laughs with Barbara Walters, trotted out onstage arm in arm with new BFF Meredith Vieira and felt an almost narcotic sense of belonging.

Despite a career characterized mainly by paralyzing self-doubt and bad, impetuous decisions to quit jobs, I began to think: I could do this. I was about to link elbows with destiny, as I had with Meredith, who, when you get close to her, smells like a combination of baby powder, lilacs and poise.

As my cab sped toward JFK to fly home to Los Angeles after taping my second episode of the popular morning chat show, producers called my agent to say I was one of their top choices. Before I'd even checked my bags curbside, we'd agreed on contractual terms.

I spent that flight envisioning my move from Los Angeles to a furnished apartment on the Upper West Side. I fantasized about the breezy rapport and private jokes I would have with the full-time driver they promised, the unpretentious but clearly expensive collection of Burberry trench coats I would acquire, and of course, the nonstop cold splash of "I told you so" my new post would throw in the faces of anyone who had doubted me. It would be hard to keep up my persona of self-deprecation with near toxic levels of smug coursing through my veins, but I would manage.

By the time I landed at LAX, I was out of the running.

The producers said not only did they want a conservative, but also, they really needed someone who was likely to get pregnant by the coming season. In the parlance of street fighters, or middle managers trying to rally their sales force after a bad quarter: It was go time. Or more specifically, it was *gonad* time.

Too bad mine were not likely to be in use anytime soon.

Just like that, I was plunged back into an obscurity so profound it made Debbie Matenopoulos look like Gwyneth Paltrow. I cried like the babies Elisabeth Hasselbeck would eventually have, endearing her not only to her bosses at *The View* but to the stay-at-home moms of America.

Sure, I can't complain. I got jobs in deep cable, on local news and in radio, and frankly any work that doesn't involve taking over my dad's automotive repair business is a blessing. But I couldn't help thinking that if I could just procreate, I would have ascended to the next level, and my gonads and I would have enjoyed the chauffeur-driven ride all the way to the middle.

It's just that, on *The View* and elsewhere, being a mommy seems to be good for business.

Babies are transformative. Yeah, they make you more loving and patient, blah blah blah, but I'm not talking about that kind of change. I'm talking about the magical baby dust that converts, say, Brooke Burke from an icy and unapproachable swimsuit model to the champion and cohost of the popularity contest *Dancing with the Stars*. Sprinkle some magic mommy dust on Angelina Jolie and she goes from knife-wielding, blood-vial-wearing, scary force of sexual energy to earth mother/goddess breast-feeding on the cover of *W* magazine.

So effective is this magic dust that it has the power to make you reconsider loathing Nancy Grace.

A Google search for the term "baby bump" yields nearly two million hits, with most of the top ten devoted to celebrity pregnancy. Think about the following babies and ask yourself how many times you've seen their lovable mugs: Ryder, Shiloh, Apple, Seraphina, Suri, Zuma, Brooklyn, and Sparrow. I used to think this was a brand-new phenomenon, that because women have increasing power and earning potential it's somehow comforting to know that we are still partially just baby-making machines. The threat we pose is mitigated by the hours we'll spend pregnant, nursing, changing diapers or otherwise tending to kiddies.

Then I read that, back in 1953, the country basically screeched to a halt to watch the birth of Little Ricky on *I Love Lucy*. A record 71.7

percent of all television-owning households tuned in, partly because the subject was still new for television, but also because the characters Lucy and Ricky were played by Lucy and Desi, who in real life were married and the parents of Desi Jr. Media coverage of the event was so massive it overshadowed the inauguration of President Eisenhower the next morning.

Cut to Demi Moore pregnant and nude on the cover of *Vanity Fair* in 1991, then to the cable sensation *The Secret Life of the American Teenager*. I guess the secret is: We even love pregnant teens! And that means you, too, Jamie Lynn Spears and Bristol Palin.

With the proliferation of media outlets (*People* magazine even has a Celebrity Baby Blog; read it to learn why pregnant Nancy O'Dell craves baked beans), we can fill the need we've always had to see the adorable little faces that result from celebrity DNA, or to observe someone known for her svelte body, like Heidi Klum or Kelly Ripa, enlarge. Entertainment news is now a nonstop "Bump Watch."

As a culture, we have a voyeuristic fascination with famous mothers, but we're simply gaga for multiples. More babies equals more babymania.

How much did we want to see the Jolie-Pitt twins, Vivienne and Knox? *People* magazine reportedly paid a record $14 million for the first photos.

Watched TLC lately?

I remember when it used to be all home decorating shows (back when I was scratching for my seat on *The View*, I used to host TLC's *While You Were Out*). Now it's mostly shows about babies and families with many, many babies, including the Duggars, who have nineteen kids with "J" names, including Jedidiah and Jinger.

Don't worry about the crazy monikers. They won't get bullied in the schoolyard because (1) Jesus loves them and (2) They are homeschooled.

Why this obsession of ours? Aside from the miracle of childbirth being inherently interesting (a living, breathing entity squirms right out of a human vagina—it never gets old!), and the thrill of seeing some tiny starlet get fat and then thin again (how Jessica Alba or Gisele Bündchen or any other celebrity lost their baby weight sells magazines every time), and the soothing sense that even our most kick-ass power women (Madonna, Katie Couric, Christina Aguilera, Sarah Jessica Parker, Michelle Obama, Hillary Clinton) had a baby yen, there is also just this: Moms are so . . . *maternal.*

Welcome to facile conjecture-ville, I hope you'll have a pleasant stay.

Mothers know things. They have superhuman strength. They are selfless, protective, gentle and sacrificing. Not *my* mother exactly—who should have named my brother and me Burden and Buzz Kill for how much she dug being a single parent—but in general, who wouldn't want to be imbued with these qualities in the eyes of the public?

Did I want to be the girl with one dead ficus and two perhaps overly adored cats? Did I want to be the woman who forgets birthdays, remembers petty grudges and drives around in an unwashed car littered with empty water bottles and crumpled scripts for jobs she didn't get?

Or could I use not only a whole new fan base, but also a wealth of new topics to mine for material?

Hell, yes.

So, I certainly didn't have a baby to help my career. But it shouldn't hurt.

one

When It Comes to Conception, Porn Is Good and *The Secret* Is Bad

*I can't let you in 'cause you're old as fuck. For this
club, you know, not for the earth.*

DOORMAN, KNOCKED UP

So, I'm thirty-eight. I'm arguably "old as fuck," and my husband and I decide it's time to pull the goalie. In the same second we decide to have a baby (after much debate, the nature of which I'll get to later), I also quietly resign myself to being infertile. I am not only "AMA" (Advanced Maternal Age; saw it written on my medical chart once and felt like Grandma Moses) but I've also had an STD, thanks to the stand-up comedian I dated for a year when I first moved to Los Angeles.

Yes, I am going to talk about the clap. Because listen, I don't want you to panic if you've had an STD or two and have seen the other side of thirty-five. Having kids later in life is the new thing, so don't sweat it.

Before the physical part of this equation, let's get into the mental part. If you have a horrible attitude, and have made the presumption, like I did, that conception is never going to happen for you, please don't be conned into thinking your crappy attitude about fertility can ruin your chances of conceiving. That seems to be the conventional wisdom tumbling out of the mouths of crypto-spiritual clowns. They try to shame you into thinking your thoughts either make you sick or heal you. In a way, it would be nice if it were that simple, but my uterus has proven that theory wrong. Way wrong.

All I did—and I did it like it was a full-time job—was worry and obsess about being infertile.

Thankfully, the uterus is impervious to "bad vibes" and the universe had bigger fish to fry than punishing me for being such a bummer with my parade of negative thoughts. *The Secret* isn't total bullshit, but in my experience, it's close.

Allow me a brief detour into both my twenties and my scarred fallopian tubes.

You first have to understand that I second-guess everything, including writing about second-guessing everything right now.

Most times I hang up the phone, I generally regret at least one thing I've said or neglected to say. When I worked in morning radio, I would spend the entire twenty-minute drive home from the studio each afternoon mulling over something idiotic I had said, like I was jamming a dull scissor into the same spot on my forearm repeatedly. After three years doing the news and being Adam Carolla's sidekick on the FM dial, this little ritual down Wilshire Boulevard improved exactly none, and even now when I record a podcast, or appear as a guest on *Dr. Phil* or some other show, I find at least one moment to kick myself in the ass about. I tell you this just so you understand how deeply I question myself, how quick I am to blame myself, and how unlikely I am to let myself off the hook for even a mild or non-existent transgression. I spend way too much of my life lightly basting in a marinade of shame.

All that being said, I refuse to be ashamed of catching chlamydia.

That's why I'm writing about it, because a bug doesn't have a personality, nor does it differentiate between nice girls and skanks. Lots of us have caught them, and it certainly doesn't mean we're dirty. There was nothing especially whorish about me; in fact, the stand-up who gave me the "lie down" was maybe my sixth sexual partner, all of whom were long-term boyfriends. It would make me feel all mysterious about things if I could spin a dark yarn detailing drunken nights with strangers, but despite the fact that my mom was a Frye boot–wearing, free love–celebrating, *Joy of Sex*–reading, laissez-faire kind of parent, I have always been kind of old-fashioned about sex. I refuse to feel like a slut even though I had the VD so bad I ended up at the free clinic in Hollywood, which is generally a sign that you are failing at life.

Even if I'd caught chlamydia from the pizza delivery guy, however, that still would not make me a bad person, and while it might rightly make you question my judgment, it seems critical to note just how common STDs are. With an estimated four million new cases of chlamydia alone occurring each year in the United States, there have to be lots of women of childbearing age who have jacked up tubes or worse. Not everyone is going to be completely forthcoming about why they have trouble getting pregnant, so you may not hear much about the clap and fertility, but I'm starting to think lots of us are in the same boat: the SS *VD*.

So, here's my story. I had never even had a yeast infection when I started having some discharge and burning in the girl parts when I was twenty-seven.

I was living down the street from a cemetery in a $385-a-month studio apartment in a building that was basically the Village of the Damned; when people asked where I lived I would either tell them travel east on Beverly until you get scared, then go about three more miles, or I would simply tell them to look for the corner of Purse Snatch and Car Jack.

My neighbors were a glamorous bunch of *bon vivants*. There was the Asian transsexual prostitute turning tricks in her studio next door to mine. There was the pudgy, middle-age dude who showed me copious poems about his cat, Shadow, his "only reason for living," and who regularly received Meals on Wheels. There was the baggy pants dude trying to be a choreographer who would play the same eight bars of "Unbreak My Heart" over and over until I wanted to Break His Face. There was the building manager, a guy on disability for chronic fatigue syndrome (Jesus, that man was tired), and there was the elderly man down the hall who rarely left his apartment but blasted every Dodger game from an old transistor radio. So this was life in the fast lane. That is, if your destination was the heart of freaking darkness.

Anyway, as you can imagine, I was uninsured, which is how I ended up getting my privates checked out by a staunch nurse with a tight blond braid at a Planned Parenthood nearby, meaning in the ghetto. She said I seemed fine, and by that, I think, she meant white; she sent me home with some yeast infection medication. Before leaving the clinic, I used the bathroom. When I went to wash my hands, I noticed the soap dispenser was empty and I remember thinking, "No soap? Doesn't soap prevent the spread of disease, and isn't that what this place is all about?"

Several visits and Pap smears later, I learned I had chlamydia, which a guy can carry and be totally asymptomatic, so I could hardly blame the comedian, although I might have felt better about the whole thing if he hadn't "all of a sudden" remembered a cocktail waitress in Charlotte who mentioned something about having something, which didn't seem relevant to mention until, um, it was.

Lots of bad medical care later, I finally went to a real doctor, who told me I had pelvic inflammatory disease from trying and failing to treat the bug with various gnarly antibiotics from the clinic.

There was such a sense of euphoria when I was being treated by an actual doctor, with a white coat and everything, that I almost didn't want to ask if there would be long-term effects, but I did and he told me my tubes might be scarred and I could have trouble having kids later. He said he didn't think so, and I asked how we would know for sure. "If you try to have kids and it doesn't work," he answered.

That was over ten years ago, but it haunts me as we commence baby making.

I take my friend, a mother of two-year-old fertility treatment twins, out for margaritas, and grill her about the entire process, taking down the name and phone number of her fertility specialist. The forty-seven-year-old redhead from Pilates who finally conceived after five attempts at in vitro fertilization, I corner her to get every detail, marveling at her determination (not to mention bankroll). When I run into a pregnant neighbor at the Coffee Bean, I trap her in a fatal talk hold while I soak up tales of daily hormone shots, Clomid cycles, acupuncture, cryopreservation of embryos and intrauterine insemination. I see her eyeing the door as her latte goes cold, but I can't let her loose.

I'm on a need-to-know basis with every woman who has ever had trouble getting pregnant. Furthermore, the girls who just flat out procreated with no trouble? I need to know their stories, too. Mainly so I can resent them. Mentally, I am socking away money for assisted reproductive technologies. I will need them all, I am certain.

Within just a few days off the pill, I am consumed with infertility and certain that because of my age and my dubious STD history it's going to be a long, barren haul that may never ever actually yield a baby. Infertility is everywhere I look until I am convinced that no one gets pregnant *just like that*, and that one-night-stand pregnancies must be an urban legend or the province of teenagers with more youthful vaginas. I walk by the newsstand, and it seems like every actress I see is either having multiples from fertility treatments or hiring a surrogate. When I think of my reproductive system, I literally picture one lonely egg, as if human eggs look like chicken eggs, covered in cobwebs and dust like Miss Havisham's wedding cake. While I'm probably supposed to be making vision boards filled with giggling babies and gloriously pregnant bellies, I'm mainly picturing that egg, decayed, rotting and old as fuck.

I start peeing on those ovulation kit sticks and trying to squeeze through the so-called fertility window. When I calculate that a day is *the optimum day*, based on half-assed knowledge cobbled together from searching the Internet and reading parts of books and unscientifically polling various women, I pressure my husband into having some very un-fun, desperate, high-strung sex the second he gets home. Afterward, I sit in bed facing the headboard with my legs elevated against the wall for twenty minutes. Someone told me this helps the swimmers succeed in getting to their destination, which may be true, but it makes you feel like a character Meg Ryan would play, bursting with such extreme quirkiness and adorable self-doubt that she's like a knife in your brain. Every morning before work, before rushing out at the ass crack of dawn to prep the morning news, I pee on a stick to find out my ovulation status. It's the least romantic, most confusing, clinical, pressure-filled month ever. I detest those sticks, the legs against the wall, the lame, forced sex.

When I get my period that first month, I am crushed. I feel about as womanly as Steve McQueen listening to a Rush song while playing Call of Duty, which is to say I feel like a total dude.

And that's when people start to quietly suggest that I am causing my own fears to come true. I should shut up about infertility and stop being so sure I won't get pregnant, because my mind is doing some voodoo on my body. *This is all my brain's fault.*

Thus I came into contact with *The Secret*, the self-help documentary that posits the "Law of Attraction," the idea that your thoughts and feelings attract events. Ostensibly, this principle is both hopeful and elegant; Oprah did two episodes on it, and I like to live according to her teachings. However, let's just say you can't master your negative thoughts. Well, too bad, because you are doing some major "manifesting" of all the disastrous bullshit that crosses your mind, or so says *The Secret* and all of the New Age-y schools of thought that run parallel.

One friend actually printed out a hundred quotes from *The Secret* for me, and I folded it and tucked it into my handbag, thinking, it can't hurt. Unless, of course, I'm found dead and I can't pretend from Beyond that I was toting that thing around with a sense of irony.

"Whatever is going on in your mind is what you are attracting," read the handout. "You become and attract what you think," it further taunted me. "People think about what they don't want and attract more of the same." And if I wasn't already filled with New Age guilt, another quote warned me, "Those who speak most of illness have illness" and "You attract your dominant thoughts."

Armed with this knowledge, I still could not stop the infertile thoughts, the ongoing calculations of how many in vitro fertilizations I could afford if I sold my condo, the image of that yellowing egg fixed in my head, burned there like an image paused too long on an early plasma TV screen. "Choose your thoughts carefully," admonished the dog-eared page of quotes. *Like I can choose my own thoughts.* I have about as much luck with this as I have with betting on horse races or corralling killer bees.

If my thoughts could have made me infertile, believe me, they would have.

After the first month of unpleasant sex and legs on the wall, I sit next to a woman at a wedding who is both a cardiologist and a new mom. She tells me, "Throw away the sticks. The sticks stress women out and cause performance problems with men. The sticks don't work. Your fertility window is three days long. Just have lots of sex, so you don't miss it. Just have Lots. Of. Sex."

Because I need structure, I ask her how much is lots, and she says every other day, to allow the Mister's sperm count to recover (I've since read this is a myth, and that every day is better, but whatever). This sounds like a plan. And while this petite woman in a fringe shawl daintily nibbling on a dinner salad isn't my doctor, she is *a* doctor, and that's good enough for me.

Even for newlyweds like us, having sex every other day, without fail, can be kind of a chore. No matter how in love you are, carefully plotted procreation flies in the face of hot sexual abandon.

That's why I always recommend porn to anyone who is trying to get pregnant.

Not only will X-rated movies increase your husband's enthusiasm for the conception process, it may also increase his fertility. In my duties as a "news" reporter, I once did a story about an evolutionary biologist at the University of Western Australia who found that looking at pornographic images of men and women together can increase the quantity and quality of a man's sperm. According to this study, watching another male having at it with a female creates a perceived "competition," thus inspiring faster, more motile swimmers. Yes, this is the kind of hard news I brought to the FM dial.

I was the Woodward and Bernstein of jizz.

It comes to me, having never actually watched porn, that I should spearhead a "let's watch porn" campaign with my husband. I had interviewed lots of porn stars while doing morning radio with Carolla, and I always thought they were sweet girls—super molested and broken, but sweet. The porn stars and their agent-boyfriends were always handing out free product, which I dutifully took home because I can't turn down free stuff, even *Sinner Takes All*.

Just about every man likes porn, and if you think yours doesn't, you are probably wrong. I once read an article in *Cosmopolitan* magazine suggesting there are four things that are true of every male: He wants to earn more than you do, he wants more oral sex, he would rather hang out with you than his buddies, and he consumes porn, whether you know it or not. Yeah, I just quoted a *Cosmo* story, which neutralizes the *Great Expectations* reference I dropped earlier, but I must say I have found those four things to be universal when it comes to guys.

"Porn and sex every other day? Um, you know, if that's what you want," says Daniel, modulating his enthusiasm for my suggestion so he doesn't seem too pervy or overeager.

For some reason, anything a married couple does just seems wholesome somehow, so I didn't bother to find this gross and I still don't.

So we delve into my stash of free DVDs. Wow. I don't know if you realize this, but there is an angry, aggressive, extreme trend in pornography right now. The drooling, spitting, pierced, tattooed adult actresses of today do lots of deliberate gagging, uncomfortable cursing, and submitting to sexual positions that can't possibly feel good unless your uncle fondled you and destroyed your ability to create personal boundaries. These girls are all penciled-in eyebrows and dry stripes of bleached hair. They are *hard*. And more to the point, they don't look like they are having any fun, which makes me wonder how any woman watching them can have any fun. Like a virgin having bad sex for the first time, I wonder what all the fuss is about. This is a multibillion-dollar industry?

That's when my husband suggests we delve into some retro porn, movies from back in the 1970s, when the women still had bush and it was all shot on film, like in *Boogie Nights*.

These foxy gals have their real boobs and the films have enough of a plot to keep me interested, 'cause I need a little something to hang my hat on, you know? Sorry to be a cliché, and I don't need it to be *The English Patient*, but I do require some kind of context for why these folks are having sex. And while I'm sure they are also molested and broken, the '70s chicks seem so much less wrathful about it. In fact, you almost get the idea most are just legit actresses working porn on the side to supplement their waitressing tips. Unlike today's jagged, crystal-meth-addicted porn stars, the actresses of yesteryear are maybe on a couple of Quaaludes, but they genuinely seem to be enjoying themselves. Feathered hair, bell-bottom jeans and round figures make them even more irresistible. We experiment with some '80s films as well, and while the production values are lower and the lace glove quotient is higher, at least you won't see today's female-boner-killing spitting and gagging.

We decide to subscribe to a service like Netflix, only for porn, which allows you to rent any two films at a time and exchange them for new ones through the mail. Then we hit the jackpot: At a hotel, we stumble across our first so-called parody porn, a graphic reimagining of *The Brady Bunch*, in which Jan engages in girl-on-girl action, Marcia pleasures herself with a dildo she keeps under her pastel bed and Alice has sex with Sam the Butcher, played by Ron Jeremy. The sets, costumes and sound track are so true to the original, you almost don't mind when an actual laugh track punctuates the dialogue. Depending on when you hit puberty, you may have had sexual thoughts about Greg or Peter, and now you get to see the whole bunch in a variety of X-rated situations, all of which manages to seem like innocent family fun. This one was so excellent, we went on to rent parodies of *Gilligan's Island*, and *Happy Days*, worth seeing for a three-way with the Fonz during which he points to graffiti on the bathroom wall that reads, "Sit on it." Surprisingly, much care is taken to avoid anachronistic tattoos, and even the lingerie is true to that era. Extra points to the casting director for finding an amazing Mr. Cunningham (he doesn't do sex scenes) and getting Ralph Malph to dye *all* of his hair red. Aaaaay.

If you're squeamish about pornography, this is a good place to start, and there are now parodies of *Seinfeld*, *The Cosby Show*, *The Office* and others. Porn parodies of hit movies have been around forever, but the sitcoms are a new twist. More laughs, more tension breakers, more Fonz.

We watch porn, we have sex every other day, I toss the ovulation sticks but desperately clutch my certainty that this whole endeavor is doomed, and oddly enough, this combination works almost immediately. In less than three months, I am pregnant.

I send out that I'm Not Fertile energy to the universe, and the universe is totally unfazed.

The Secret is all fine and good until it blames you for a little— okay, an excessive—amount of worry. I feel for couples who can't conceive, who go through months and even years of expensive, grueling invasive treatments that make them feel like losers, and I would hate for anyone to truly believe their own gloomy thoughts are the cause of their troubles. That's why I tell you that while I am a statistical sampling of one, I have personally debunked the Law of Attraction insofar as it pertains to the functionality of reproductive organs. It doesn't matter what the hell you're thinking; if you are having lots of sex and there is nothing medically wrong with you, if your body is ready, you can't think your way out of a fertilized egg.

The real secret is this: The universe is random and unpredictable and chaotic. Meditate on that.

two

(You're) Having My Baby,
or Anka Management

My husband knows I'm pregnant before I do, because of salmon and popcorn. One I eat to excess, one I throw across the room.

After ingesting a huge hunk of salmon for dinner at the restaurant down the street, I bring home leftovers and chow them down for breakfast the next day. Around noon, I declare that I will need to go back to that same corner bistro for the salmon again, which I scarf down with some asparagus and capellini. I have leftovers for both breakfast and lunch the following day. That's five straight meals consisting mainly of salmon.

Something seems fishy.

Since I was eight years old and realized that bacon was basically Wilbur from *Charlotte's Web*, I've been mostly a vegetarian. For lack of a more nuanced way of putting it, meat grosses me out and I can rarely eat animal flesh without thinking of gnawing away on a creature that was once mooing, swimming, or doing whatever it is chickens do. For that reason, I eat fish rarely and, if I do, order it well done and with a side of yucky face. Aside from which, it's my philosophy that if you're going to binge, if you want to lose yourself through the low-risk–high-shame vice of overeating, you go either crunchy (box of Snyder's pretzels, fistfuls of tortilla chips) or sweet (any offering from a Whitman's Sampler excluding the Cherry Cordial). You don't waste valuable calories on something rife with protein and nutrients, but instead you look for a certain yummy, comforting jejuneness.

As for the popcorn, instead of cramming it down my salmon-hole, I throw a bowl of it across the room at my husband, having lost my temper during a fight I pick over nothing.

Before the bowl even lands, I'm ashamed and confused. I thought my days of uncontrolled temper tantrums were over. I've thrown lots of things in my time, hitting rage bottom the day I almost got arrested for spraying a $26 tube of self-tanner on the door of a spa that refused to exchange it.

See, they sold me "dark" instead of "light" and really should have taken it back or exchanged it, but the spa lady gave me a lot of attitude and a flat, snotty refusal, after which I left in a huff, slammed the door with a few insults about her customer service skills, and sprayed the door with the entire tube of offending "dark" tanner. It's the kind of idiotic, out-of-control, petty moment you are glad no one has witnessed, until of course the spa lady tracks down your number and calls to tell you not only has the outburst been witnessed, it's been captured by security cameras. She threatened to press charges for vandalism. I apologized profusely, made a lame joke about bronzing her door and offered to pay for any damages. I did this not only to avoid court, but because I was genuinely in the wrong. I hung up and vowed never to lose my shit—in public *or* private—over nothing ever again, because even if you don't get busted, your conscience is like a security camera that picks up every angle, records your worst moments and logs them with brutal detail.

The hormonal popcorn tossing, along with the sudden, obsessive salmon-eating, tips off my husband that I'm not quite myself.

After work, my husband stops by the drugstore for a home pregnancy test. My period is not late, and I know the test, like my outlook, will not be positive.

I pee on the stick, floss and brush my teeth to kill some time while it soaks and almost forget about the white plastic stick teetering on the edge of the sink. Two pink lines. This can't be right. I pee on the other stick. Two pink lines. I read the instructions again, knowing the Mister is wondering what is taking so long. Two pink lines means we did it. *We did it.* I think about coming up with some clever way of telling him, something we'll always remember and can tell the child over and over until he's sick of the story. Now I'm really taking forever in the bathroom trying to conjure something magical. My mind is both racing and blank. I got nothing.

I just casually walk over to my husband sitting on the couch and show him the stick.

We grab each other and I start cackling, or more accurately, I toggle between a creepy, not-totally-appropriate-to-the-situation guffaw and making an Edvard Munch *The Scream* face. There is a chorus of "holy shit" and "oh my god" and we both don't know quite what to do, or what this means to our ability to spend money on flat-screen televisions and overpriced Sunday morning omelets. We take a picture of the stick, and of me posing next to it, neither of which comes out; the stick is unreadable (and so is my face, though strained and greasy are easy adjectives). Those tests just don't photograph well. On the other hand, because this idea doesn't turn out to be very original, I later notice that every pregnancy blog on the Web features the very same photo, positive pregnancy test sticks captured with perfect clarity, so chalk that up as our first parental failure. And my pregnancy has gotten off to a start that is not only out of focus, but hacky.

The next morning is just like any other, except it's four thirty a.m. and I'm pregnant.

As I'm fumbling around for a couple of tablets of folic acid to down with my herbal tea and grabbing a protein bar to eat in the car on the way to the studio, I hear Paul Anka and Odia Coates belting out their number-one hit from 1974, "(You're) Having My Baby," which my husband downloaded the night before and is blasting through our apartment. It was a favorite of Adam Carolla, who once spent half of our morning show breaking down the lyrics. If you're looking for a romantic tune about procreating with vague references to abortion, this is your song. It starts out fine: "Havin' my baby, what a lovely way of sayin' how much you love me" before it turns into something creepy: "Didn't have to keep it, wouldn't put you through it. You could have swept it from your life but you wouldn't do it. No, you wouldn't do it." Oddly enough, that wasn't even the controversial part of the tune. At the time, there was a feminist outcry against the song's seemingly sexist tone, specifically the possessive pronoun "my." To this day, when playing the song live, Anka sings "having *our* baby."

Daniel and I belt out the original chorus together ("Havin' my baby. You're a woman in love and I love what's goin' through you") and he hands me a CD of the song, which I listen to the entire way to work, on a loop.

Months before, we'd gone on a weekend getaway to Avila Beach, a small town in San Luis Obispo County just a couple of hours northwest of Los Angeles, basically a poor man's Santa Barbara. On the agenda: (1) Get some clam chowder in one of those sourdough bread bowls; (2) Get close to the seals on the pier; and (3) Figure out whether or not to have a baby.

On our way back from doing the first two, we walked about two miles from a cheesy glass-bottom restaurant docked in the ocean back to our hotel, a dodgy mom and pop that smelled of mildewed bathing suits and sour buttermilk with top notes of ass. As we walked on the curvy, friable highway along the shore, we tackled the biggest question of our newlywed lives: Is having a kid an inspirational gift or a dream-crushing burden?

Just like I didn't want a big wedding, because giant parties and tiered wedding cakes have no meaning for me personally and I didn't want to be sucked into the culture's pricey rituals, I wanted to make sure having kids wasn't just falling prey to society's biggest con job. For those of us who aren't baby crazy, who didn't grow up around babies, who saw babysitting only as an easy way to steal beer and make free long-distance phone calls, to those of us who see ourselves first as worker bees and achievers and not sweet-voiced nurturers who can't wait to decorate a nursery and laminate ultrasound photos, this kid thing was in no way a slam dunk.

There is a paranoid part of me that always thinks I'm being conned, and that wants to watch my back to stay one step ahead of The Man. So we tried to tackle the decision from a practical standpoint, methodically reviewing pros and cons.

First we brainstormed the cons. Kids are expensive, consume your time, make it hard to travel to random beach towns because you feel like it . . . and create a whole new level of fear. I get nauseous just thinking about what could happen to my dad riding his bicycle on the way to work. When I was a lifeguard as a teenager, while the other guards secretly drank rum from giant plastic cups, I sat slathered in zinc worrying that some kid was going to drown on my watch and I would die a slow death of regret and melanoma. I'm a worrier, and I worried about how much I would worry. Just seeing a prepubescent boy on a skateboard makes my mind shriek, *Careful, kid! You are one Hostess wrapper from a broken femur. Or a persistent vegetative state.*

Having a child opens you up to all kinds of emotional liabilities.

With the hotel coming into view, or maybe we were just smelling it, we came up with the pros. It would seem sort of sad to be in our fifties and sixties with no kids, no homey pictures on our desks at work, no college dorms to visit, no grandkids. It could be fun to mix our genes, see how the recombination turns out. It might be nice to have built-in caretakers when we're old, someone to wax my mustache in my twilight years and make fun of Daniel's old-man ear hair and perhaps feed us rice pudding by hand. And it might be sweet to shift our focus from ourselves, and liberating to live in the sloppy mess of parenthood instead of hustling for the next work-related validation.

The most pressing pro is something I struggled to articulate, but which I've always thought of in terms of a giant menu that you get when you pull up a chair at the table of life.

There isn't much on it.

When it comes to experiences that are Big, the menu is limited, less like an IHOP and more like the entrée options at a catered function. You can move to a new city, fall in love, follow your dream—or have kids. Maybe I'm missing a couple, but the kitchen is limited and if you wait too long, they run out of things. I'm not exactly the kind of girl who came up with baby names in elementary school and rocked her dollies to sleep. I envy women who love babies, who know just how to hold them and comfort them, have always known. I was not that girl. Still, if having babies is the life-altering, perspective-giving, kick-ass miracle that people say it is, why would we want to miss out on one of the few peak experience entrées on the universe's menu?

I'm a sucker for research, for polling everyone I know about every decision I make, but could anyone really give us a straight answer? Once you have kids, you can hardly admit it's a sham; you're in too deep. However, one thing struck us as we headed to our hotel room in Avila Beach: If parenthood truly sucked, no one would have more than one child, and the vast majority of couples do just that. This seemed the weightiest evidence of all.

That was it.

We were 51 percent sure we wanted to have kids. Procreating won by a slim margin, but a W is a W. We were back to the hotel and had put a mint on the pillow of our future, or maybe a turd, but we were willing to chance it.

So, I head into work with the Paul Anka song in my head and this hugest of all secrets in my heart and uterus, just wanting to grab every single person and tell them the news. The plot that was hatched that day at the beach is in full flower. *"I'm a woman in love and I love what it's doin' to me. Having my baby."*

three

Inner Child, Meet New Baby, Please Don't Smother It

Being pregnant for the first time, I'm scared and I want my mommy. I just don't want *my* mommy.

My mom hates kids, always has. She didn't put her cigarette out on my arm or throw me in a pit of snakes, but having kids just wasn't her diaper bag, and it showed.

I'm not here to trash my mother, only to worry that I'll become her.

While most people say having children gives them new compassion for their parents, I'm not having that experience so far. Instead, I'm filled with a renewed, fuming and bottomless discontent about the mom hand I was dealt, which consisted of one truly evil, now fortunately dead, stepmother, and a wildly superior though still problematic biological mom, who raised me with a combination of ambivalence and benign neglect.

For her part, it was nothing personal against me. She just found all babies to be life-snatching bummers.

The syllogism was as impossible to ignore as a tot shrieking in a high chair, spitting noodles: Mom hates children. I am a child. Therefore, mom hates me. I must be quite an irritating burden. In fact, I grew up thinking that everyone hates babies. It was all I knew.

Don't get me wrong. My mom is a fun person, and people genuinely like her. If Auntie Mame were less chirpy, more medicated, and prone to dating angry, homeless Berkeley poets or leaving her kids for a month to chop trees in Vermont, that would be my mom. Part Mame, part maimed, all out of her element when it came to lullabies and hugs.

To this day, if a baby cries in a restaurant with my mom around, we all have to bail immediately, but not before she shoots the family several piercing, withering looks. Long looks. She doesn't look away until she has properly shamed the parents for ruining her meal and her day. When she hears a baby cry—or, frankly, gurgle, laugh or even sing—she fixes her face in an expression to communicate to the world that she is being put upon, that the sounds coming from *your* child are no less than an ice pick in her temporal lobe.

I am not her, or she, or however you say it. I know that, but there are tinges of her intolerance, times I notice my head involuntarily snapping toward a howling baby in a restaurant, a vestige of that adhesive notion that babies are serenity-piercing killjoys.

I'm terrified that just as I have her broad shoulders and wide feet, I may inherit her lackluster mothering skills. How can I be sure I won't resent my baby? My therapist assures me I won't, that true maternal detachment of my mother's sort is very rare, that even though my baby is only partially cooked, I'm already bonded to the kid, and that seems true. Still, when I think about how much the whole experience sucked for my mom, I worry.

My mother's exasperation with me started even before I was born.

She bought "It's a Boy" cards when she was pregnant, just trying to sway the gender gods. Her desire for a second boy was based on this chestnut: "A boy would be your father's problem." This story isn't one she tried to hide. In fact, it was in heavy rotation on the "Mom's hilarious anecdote Top 40," staying there for an unprecedented twenty years, right up there with predicting my brother would never pass the bar (he did, on the first try) and falling asleep during one of my particularly boring ballet recitals.

Mom's bouquet of crazy sometimes has top notes of mean with a strong insensitivity finish.

"If you look at pictures, your mom holds you like a sack of potatoes, like she didn't connect. I think she must have had that postpartum thing," says my dad, trying to explain some of this, trying to defend her even though they have been divorced since I was three. He argues that it wasn't her fault; she just wasn't cut out for motherhood. In one old snapshot taken in a park somewhere, she holds me as I hold my stuffed bunny, my older brother is down at her feet, and she is looking away, yellow headband in her black hair, squinting. If there was a caption, it might read, "How can I get the fuck out of this?"

When I was a few months old, she got a job as a Los Angeles County school bus driver so she could afford to pay a nanny named Inez to babysit me for the first two years of my life. Let that sink in for a sec: My mother, a college graduate with an above-genius IQ, who could do Rain Man stuff like counting cards, preferred spending her days driving a diesel school bus through the smog-choked San Fernando Valley over staying home with her kids.

When I was three and my brother five, she decided she needed a break from the whole married-with-kids endeavor and left the family for six months to take a job in Chicago. By the time she got back, she was starting to get that "you're not such a good mom" look from people, including the judge, who awarded custody of my brother and me to my dad.

His wife, however, suggested I would be better off with my mom, and that's how I ended up with her, in a flat in San Francisco. Most of the time, anyway.

Once a month, starting when I was four, she put me on a plane alone to see my dad back in L.A. That isn't even legal anymore; kids that young can't fly unaccompanied. Summers and holidays, she put me on a Greyhound bus to stay with my grandparents in Santa Barbara. Those were ten-hour bus rides, just one little girl reading *Mad* magazine and eating Twizzlers with an assortment of vagrants, fugitives and visitors to the California Men's Colony. When I confronted my mom about it, she asked, "What was I supposed to do? Drive you myself all those times?"

Um . . . yes?

Back at home during the school year, I spent up to four hours a day on public buses and streetcars, to and from school, to and from ballet, to and from Sunday school. Four nights a week after ballet class, I would trudge to the bus stop in front of a tranny bar with a bun in my hair and a giant book bag across my chest. To get to my bus stop, I would walk past a row of double-parked cars, parents awaiting their daughters. On rainy days I begged my mother to pick me up, but she never did. It didn't dawn on me to feel sorry for myself until much later, but I've sure as hell made up for it since. When I go back to San Francisco, I visit that corner of Church and Market like I can flag down that little girl in her bun and leg warmers and scoop her out of the wind.

My childhood best friend, Amy, lived a couple of blocks away with her "two moms," who celebrated their anniversary every year with a lavender cake. These people seemed like gay Doris Days living in Pleasantville compared to the chaos at my place.

When Amy came over, we would order pizza and antipasto from Haystack Pizza (I still know the number by heart) and scarf it down while my mom disappeared into her room. To amuse ourselves, we would walk across the thick shag carpet in the living room and count the fleas that landed on our ankles. Mom wasn't exactly a stellar home-maker, and aside from the emotional mess, the place was usually un-kempt, with dirty pots on the stove for days, unpaid bills and junk mail teetering in high piles throughout the house and a cat box that was cleaned at long and irregular intervals.

Once, Amy and I were sitting around the kitchen table with my mom after school (Synergy, an elementary school without walls or desks where we called our teachers "Dusty" and "Cindy" and rarely bothered with things like geography and fractions) when the word "cervix" came up. I don't remember how, but it was San Francisco in the '70s and peo-ple spoke about sexuality pretty freely.

Ten-year-old Amy responded with some obvious naïveté about the cervix, which prompted my mother to lean toward her in an ex-plosion of incredulity and snap, "It's *your body*. It's your vagina. Stick your finger in there and feel around!"

Granted, this may have been sound advice. In fact, Amy says she has since suggested female friends of hers with a seeming lack of self-awareness and ownership of their bodies do the same. At the time, though, like most interactions with my mother, it was intimidating and freaky. While the overall message may have been a good one— get to know your own body; don't have vagina shame—Mom was incapable of calibrating it for her audience and, moreover, unwilling to bother. She didn't have a clue why this would rattle us, still can't see herself as others see her, doesn't give a shit, really, which is part of her charm but was also massively disturbing to a daughter. I didn't appreciate my mother barking at my elementary school chum to stick her finger in her vagina.

Eccentric, quirky and boundary-crossing are great qualities in, say, the neighbor on a sitcom, but not in a parent.

Because she spent the bulk of her energy just trying to escape motherhood, either so she could go out folk dancing with her friend Maureen or shut the door to her room and watch a small black-and-white TV, it was jarring when her notable and abiding absence was punctuated by moments of extreme presence. The pattern made me really nervous throughout most of my childhood, because I never knew when she would shift from completely tuned out to right in my face, or my friend's face, telling us to get into our cervixes.

She didn't have any middle gears.

It still makes me cringe, and recall those years as one long, rolling, gnawing wave of dread.

When she saw a couple of girls picking on me at a Synergy School function she attended, she cornered Amy, as a representative of this group, and probably the only girl she knew by name, and yelled, "Do you know what you're doing to her? She is devastated by how you girls are acting."

It was terrifying the way my mother defended me. And confusing. She didn't want my little friends to treat me like an outcast, but she had no problem sending me off by myself on a Greyhound bus, a far more dangerous experience for which she regularly volunteered me. When my brother stayed with us one weekend a month, she would rip the head off anyone who bullied him, a kid she lost custody of for ditching, a kid she wasn't even raising. We were everything and we were nothing.

Still, she is not and was not a bad person. In the end, she lacked social graces and was operating way outside of her skill set, but she was not malicious.

Here's where I struggle to say something positive so I don't come across like a horrible, ungrateful daughter just for telling the truth. The more self-reliant we became, the more tolerant she was, and I can say she did have some sparkling mom moments.

Every summer, she would take us to a family camp in Yosemite, where she would mainly work on her tan and leave us to fend for ourselves. At night, however, she would read to us by flashlight, one chapter before bed, usually Vonnegut or Steinbeck. The year she read us *Of Mice and Men*, we couldn't wait until sundown, to hear our mother's voice, low and deliberate, tell the story of Lennie and George and their dream about tending rabbits and living off the fat of the land. I still think my mother has the most perfect voice in the world, can still hear her clear diction, the sound of mosquitoes buzzing and paperback pages turning in the darkness. When George shot Lennie, we were decimated for days. This should be in the bad memory pile, and perhaps linger only as evidence that Mom should have stuck to age-appropriate literature. Instead, getting caught up in that story was like being tucked into a sleeping bag, tight, inescapable and cozy.

Books were holy to my mother, as were plays, musicals and the ballet, all of which she dragged me to throughout my childhood, toting me along to everything from *Annie* to *Richard II*. If there was a band of Slavic folk dancers in town, we saw them. If a slapdash improv troupe was giving a never-ending performance in the Mission District, we were there. I was generally the only kid at revivals of Judy Garland movies at the Castro Theatre and poetry readings at Sacred Grounds, the coffee shop my mom owned in Haight-Ashbury. On the way to these outings, she always seemed flustered and quiet (the time I lost my patent leather shoe and made us twenty minutes late to *The Nutcracker*, she didn't talk to me for days) and, frankly, pretty bored by my company. Again, if you don't like kids but have to live with one, even evenings spent at enriching cultural events of your choosing are like bad dates you just have to get through so you can go home, wipe off your makeup, unhook your uncomfortable bra, and relax. Still, she communicated that being creative wasn't something frivolous, but instead that artists were contributing something deeply important to society.

My mother was a true patron of the arts.

This is how we came to house a poet named Max, who lived in our garage for about seven years rent-free. He sauntered upstairs to use our bathroom and do his laundry, but otherwise spent most of his time on a dilapidated plastic lawn chair on the sidewalk outside of our place, where he was prone to breaking out into freestyle verse. He wore an army jacket and was freakishly tall and rail thin, thanks to constant juice fasts. His teeth were like piano keys, some permanently depressed, and I dreaded running into him on my way home, especially if I had to explain to a friend why there was a giant (literally) starving artist snapping his fingers and rhyming in our driveway.

I wished every single day that he would leave, didn't care about his huge following in Europe, just wanted to have a freak-free childhood for a while. If I could say one positive thing about Max's long stay, it is only in retrospect. I couldn't articulate it at the time, but our garage poet was a manifestation of my mother's abiding sense that art was valuable, something to be supported and cultivated.

Even though parenthood seemed a dismal experience, I knew nothing made my mother happier than when I was artistic. Okay, I was a terrible visual artist, and when I brought home a lopsided ceramic ashtray or drippy watercolor painting, she would pretty much mock me and toss them or shove them in a dresser drawer with a pile of old scarves. But however much she disdained my crappy crafts, she paid for those ballet lessons for years without complaint and she always encouraged me to write, something she probably regrets right about now.

I knew she meant it when she said she liked some essay or book report I brought home, because she was incapable of sugarcoating. Although when I think about it, sugarcoating is sort of what moms are for, and I could have used some of that. But I got what I got and sometimes I'm at peace with that and other times I'm sad for what I missed.

I married a man whose mother is appropriate, dresses well, says the right things and has personalized stationery. This is no accident.

Of course, like everyone who tries to correct the things their parents got wrong, I will endeavor never to humiliate my child (*knock wood, if I am lucky enough to actually have one*) by being super weird or saying tactless things, but there is a strong chance I will fail at least some of the time.

My prime screw-up-the-kid years are far off, though; it's really the baby thing that concerns me now, the looming possibility that tending to an infant will be at best thankless and boring, at worst a stifling slow death, a suffocation by talc-scented swaddle. If I am truly my mother's daughter, there is the possibility that before I make my child miserable in ways he will recall, he will make me miserable, just by existing, just by being a tiny bundle of needs.

My therapist says I am at "high risk" for postpartum depression, because of all of what went down with my own mother. She calls in my husband for a joint session, lets him know he will have to look for warning signs and be prepared to toss some Prozac down my gullet if I get all withdrawn and affectless. If this happens, I'm assured that it will pass quickly. As we sit there on her couch holding hands, I like the way we must look to her: happy, respectful of each other, in love, and we aren't faking it for her sake. It isn't often I feel like a show-off for anything to do with my sanity, but the best thing I could do for a child, choose a father who is warm and stable and solid, I have already done. And I want my fucking gold star. And I think I see it glinting in my therapist's eyes. My man is good daddy material, and she knows it.

(Hopefully, it's not too Woody Allen that I write about my therapist. When you're as mental as I am, having struggled with everything from paralyzing stage fright to various existential career crises and bouts of crippling loneliness, therapists are important in your life.)

At the moment, I don't communicate with my mother at all, haven't spoken to her in about a year. It's not uncommon for me to take mom breaks when she gets to be too much, because while *you* might feel too guilty to cut your mom off, I don't have that problem.

I don't owe her anything.

She kept me alive for eighteen years, and while I appreciate that, she did it with such a minimum of effort and aptitude that it sometimes feels like our exchange in this lifetime is complete. She mostly phoned in being a mother and now I phone in being a daughter, which is to say I don't phone her at all. Oddly enough, she would love me to call her every day, like my brother does; fill her in. I think this is because she is bored and the comings and goings of our lives as adults are interesting, in stark contrast to the misshapen ceramic ashtrays and poopy diapers of our childhoods. I get it. Now that I can wipe my own ass and don't require full-time un-fun care, I'm a real hoot. But I'm also a resentful, grudge-holding hoot with "Cat's in the Cradle" playing in my head on a loop.

Before going ahead with the baby making, I ran all of this by my therapist, who did the best thing a therapist has ever done, and I've had a lot of them. She offered me $1 million if I have a baby and don't love it. She's that positive I'm going to be okay.

She helps me make a plan to get some help for the first few weeks after the baby so I don't get too sleep-deprived, hire a night nurse to do what some more capable mothers do for their daughters, help out with the bathing and swaddling and midnight comforting, model nurturing behavior, tell me everything is going to be okay.

The rest is just faith.

I am working on this chapter at a diner when a baby starts wailing and chucking Cheerios from a paper bowl. It's not a beautiful sound to me, but I force myself to question whether it's the worst, or whether an even more festering sound is my mother's voice in my head; not reading great literature, but her own flawed script about motherhood.

four

Pregatory

If purgatory is a temporary state of suffering, pregatory is a three-month no-man's-land during which your soul lurks between being an expectant mom and being who you were before.

They say you can't be "a little bit pregnant," but that's exactly what you are at first, when you don't feel or look any different. You're the same, but you're utterly changed.

You aren't supposed to say anything to anyone about your baby, because for weeks and weeks what may or may not be your child is just a sac of yolk without so much as a heartbeat.

Partially, keeping your mouth shut is pragmatic, because whomever you tell, you will have to un-tell if the pregnancy doesn't stick. And partially, it's just being superstitious. I knock wood so many times my knuckles bleed.

Here's how it sounds when I talk to my husband:

We can send the baby to the school around the corner, I mean, you know, knock on wood, if everything is okay. I hope the baby has blue eyes even though I have brown eyes, you know, knock wood, if the baby has eyes. *We should probably be trying to find a pediatrician for the baby, if, knock wood, we actually have the baby. Let's try to get a secondhand crib; the baby won't know the difference. I mean, knock wood, if we have one* (followed by the weird addition of knocking on my forehead in case the surface is not actually wood but some sort of IKEA-based wood product that would not have the persuasive powers of actual wood).

I'm feeling very self-conscious about all my OCD wood knocking until I read that a couple of psychologists came up with the concept of "availability bias," a brain quirk that makes us inclined to wildly overestimate the probability of events associated with memorable occurrences.

Even if an event is rare, if it's memorable, it becomes more available in our minds and thus seems more common, like plane crashes and child abductions.

The minute I read about this theory, it immediately explains not only my sense that the entire population has fertility problems, but also my feeling that all women lose at least three pregnancies in the first trimester. Vivid tales of miscarriages are so available in my mind, it's as though no pregnancy has ever gone the distance. This one's sister-in-law had four miscarriages and that one's cousin started bleeding at the grocery store and lost her baby, and this one has a compromised cervix and a poorly shaped uterus . . . the horrific stories take center stage in my mind, linking arms in a kick line, glittering in gold leotards, blinding me with a show-stopping, heartbreaking, attention-grabbing, relentless song and dance.

A throng of people in line at Starbucks, a swarm of drivers vying for a spot in the Trader Joe's parking lot, a crush of humanity at a downtown sample sale, I dispense with all of this proof that human beings are having no trouble reproducing themselves and decide instead that it's a wonder any of us made it out alive at all and I should follow the common practice and keep the pregnancy mum for twelve weeks.

This is the hardest secret I've ever kept, so I constantly fantasize about telling people, about telling everyone.

This is followed by mentally rehearsing how I will disclose losing the baby. Will I even use the phrase "lost the baby" or just keep it clinical, tell them I "miscarried" with a brief medical explanation and a sunny sign-off about how we'll try again next month? Will I send out a group e-mail, subject line: "sad news"? Or maybe I'll have my husband roll the miscarriage calls, while I sit next to him listening and quietly weeping, turning a lamp on and off like Glenn Close in *Fatal Attraction*. Of course, in this mental rehearsal, we are always perched in a cozy nursery, which makes the vision even more poignant, because I'm sitting against a freshly painted, pale yellow wall on a nursing rocker I won't be needing with a couple of sad little plush toys on my lap. My pregnancy hormones are like an endocrinological remote control, constantly switching the channel in my brain to Lifetime.

"Are your boobs sore?" asks my friend Lucy, who has three kids and used to be the anchor of the morning news show where I worked as a field reporter.

"Yes. Very sore," I answer.

"You're pregnant," she says decisively. "Trust me. You're still pregnant."

I have long chats with her on the phone while she puts on her makeup to anchor the evening news in Houston and I stroll endlessly around the block asking a million questions about pregnancy and knowing that I won't have to un-tell her if I miscarry, she will simply know, because she is one of these women who seem to have magical mommy powers. And this is the beginning of something I will feel throughout, a kinship with anyone who has a baby. I'm in the club; just barely and maybe not for keeps, but I'm in the club.

Lucy is the only person I tell, before I even get the official results from the blood test my doctor takes. Well, the only friend. I yap about being pregnant to any and all strangers, valets, waitresses, and salesclerks because I will never see them again and won't need to un-tell them. And I love saying it, finding ways to jam it into any conversation.

Waitress: "Welcome, can I get you a drink?"

Me: "I wish I could order a cocktail, but you know . . . I'm *pregnant.* So what would be a good drink for someone *in my condition? Which is pregnant?*

Dry Cleaner: "Your shirts will be ready Thursday."

Me: "Oh, great. That's perfect, because I want to wear these shirts while they still fit, because I'm getting bigger. Because I'm *pregnant.* So, see you Thursday. I'll be the pregnant one, in case I lose my ticket."

Lady in line at bagel shop: "I think you were ahead of me."

Me: "Oh, gosh, thanks so much. I'm so hungry these days, because I'm *pregnant.*"

Valet: "Garage closes at midnight."

Me: "I'm *pregnant.*"

Non sequiturs will do when you really can't work it in organically. It becomes this secret between me, my husband, my fetus, my doctor and any service industry professional or stranger who gives me twelve seconds of their time. It reminds me of using a fake name when I was a teenager hanging out at the arcade at Fisherman's Wharf in San

Francisco, where I grew up. That person, "Andi," was my much cooler alter ego; she was a B-cup, thanks to a stuffed bra, and had a fictional bio, complete with married parents who lived in Pacific Heights and who were both college professors. Likewise, this anonymous first trimester version of myself, this character I play for strangers, is nothing like me; she is so sure about the health of her baby she never knocks wood, wouldn't even know what that meant. She is carefree and psyched. She's planning on delivering at home with a midwife, maybe squatting on one of those plastic yoga balls in a candlelit room filled with sage and confidence in Mother Nature.

On the other hand, despite being "a little bit pregnant," too little to openly discuss, it's all I can think about. It dictates every morsel I put in my mouth, every Google search in my computer, every thought and daydream in my head.

The "tri" in first trimester should really be spelled "try," as in, try not to tell people even though you can't believe they don't know just by looking at you. While self-absorption isn't one of the standard pregnancy symptoms, it is certainly pervasive in my case. Since it is all about me, and the totally unique miracle that I am creating a new life, I can't fathom how my coworkers at the radio station don't notice that I've swapped my coffee for tea, that I'm practically wearing a bikini to do the news every day because my inner thermostat is all screwed up and I'm standing there shuffling papers in a flop sweat. The studio, like every room, feels like a sauna I'm standing in fully clothed.

How can they not notice that I'm constantly adjusting the air conditioner to try and cool off the studio every single commercial break? I become very conscious of the packets of Wheat Thins and baggies full of pretzels on my console, the crumbs from countless Fig

Newtons, a dead giveaway of my new morning eating schedule, which is constant. There are now blotting papers next to my laptop for the slicks of oil that form on my cheeks by nine thirty a.m.

The "try" could also stand for "try" not to feel nauseous and ravenous, the twin symptoms that have overtaken my body. These twins go everywhere together and even dress alike. The nausea makes me hungry, the food I eat to settle my stomach makes me queasy, and the twins make me gain an obscene amount of weight in the first three months.

Whining about gaining weight makes me feel about as cutting edge and literary as a Cathy cartoon, but this is a pregnancy book, so *aaack*! My inner critic can suck it.

Morning sickness doesn't hit in the morning, but any time of day and especially in the late afternoon, and it doesn't make me throw up, which might be nice because I wouldn't be gaining about six times the recommended amount for the first trimester if I did toss some of the calories back up. The nausea I feel can only be described as a motion sickness so intense it feels like I rode in the back of an old station wagon, while reading, to an amusement park, where I rode the spinning teacups for an hour before returning home by helicopter through choppy weather to my houseboat lit only by a flickering, fluorescent disco ball. When it hits, all I want is a giant sack of cheese crackers to make it go away.

Anything tangy calls to me: oranges, peaches, lemonade, vinegar, cherry yogurt. Protein bars become appetizers for meals consisting of other protein bars. I fall asleep with a spoon in my hand, a half-empty bowl of oatmeal congealing on the nightstand. I wake up, spoon still in hand, and finish it. It's difficult to separate a true craving, which you are supposed to satisfy because it means your body must require some nutrient therein, from the sense that I must eat just a little bit of everything in case my baby needs it, will starve without it, will somehow be deficient because of my unwillingness to eat a handful of peanuts or a can of tuna. The strongest craving I have is for Guinness beer—not just any beer, but something dark and viscous—which I want to drink with a mustard-covered soft pretzel. This is bizarre because I've never even tasted Guinness, though I served it to many a table as a waitress. It must have been the mumbo jumbo I read online about Irish beer containing iron.

I don't give in to the beer, but each time I walk by the Drawing Room, a dive bar down the block from my house, I pause and wonder why I didn't take full advantage of drinking when I could, why I didn't while away afternoons in that cool dark guzzling stout on a bar stool patched with duct tape. Anyway, who cares what the hell food and drink I want to ingest while pregnant? Just know I want a lot of it.

I'm going to complain a bit more for a second, before I apologize for complaining, so please humor me.

There is also a burning sensation in my heart, and I can't figure out what it is, before I put together that a burning in my heart area could be a thing I've heard about called "heartburn."

There is my first hemorrhoid, concurrent with and certainly related to niggling bouts of constipation. There are leg cramps, concurrent with and certainly related to nightly insomnia, both of which I treat by spending hours in the middle of the night sitting in the bathtub listening to podcasts of *This American Life* and staring at my belly poking up above the water. There is something my dermatologist calls "an estrogen surge," which results in cystic acne on my chin and jawline and most frustratingly across my chest, because what good is having cleavage for the first time when you can't showcase it because even when covered by concealer, it is lumpy and odd-looking?

"Overactive sebaceous glands on your neck," whispers my hairdresser, as he shampoos my hair, and the accidental shaming takes me back to my teen years, during which I had terrible skin and some-times took a "me" day off from school if there was an especially bad breakout I couldn't hide.

While I wasn't pregnant during those years, I certainly looked like it thanks to the chub I acquired when I quit ballet and started soft serve. In fact, the headmaster of my high school called me into his office my sophomore year to let me know he had heard I was preg-nant, and to tell me with studied, "I'm-an-educator" compassion that he "was there for me" if I needed help. I assured him I was not preg-nant, could not be, as I was a virgin, to which he replied with obvious disbelief, "Okay, but if you need to talk, I'm here." I stared at his gray crew cut and squinted my eyes before repeating that I was not, in fact, with child. "Right, but if you need to talk, it would be totally between us." At a highfalutin prep school, I guess a puffy, carb-eating Jew on scholarship was basically Claireece Precious Goddamn Jones. No baby would be born to me that year, but an eating disorder was already crawling by then. Thanks, Mr. Butler. Maybe you meant well, or maybe you were just a do-gooding jerk who couldn't tell the differ-ence between fat and pregnant.

So, anyway, it doesn't feel good to have pimples on my neck so glaring as to trigger Butler flashbacks, but at least it gives me an ex-cuse to say, "Oh, yeah. It's an estrogen surge. I'm not supposed to say anything yet, but *I'm pregnant*," using a stage whisper and kind of hoping the whole salon overhears so they can make a fuss over me.

There are Sea-Bands on my wrists, stupid acupressure things you buy at the drugstore for motion sickness, and I'm always chewing on ginger candies from the health food store to tamp down the nausea. Though neither works at all, they make me feel closer to the pregnant side of limbo. After all, each day, each hour, I wonder if I'm still pregnant and I have only my burgeoning acne and gripping vertigo to tell me, yes, I am.

At Oscar time, I am hired to make jokes on the red carpet with my cohost on the deep cable talk show I've been doing for a couple years. The makeup artists have to shade my face, even my nose, which is widening. Although the wardrobe lady begs me to get at least two Mystic Tans before the event, I can't, because they might be toxic, so I show up so pale Nicole Kidman and Amy Adams make Casper jokes to my face (I didn't actually interview either of them, but you get the idea—I was white). My feet get swollen and blistered on the red carpet, my skin is a mess with no faux tan to cover it, I'm sure everyone has noticed my puffy belly and beefy upper arms, and the mental energy I should be using to plan my "off the cuff" remarks I mostly spend finding ways to get back to the craft services table so I can pick the fried noodles off a giant pan of Chinese chicken salad.

Here's the thing about pregnancy complaining: I feel terrible about it. It makes me uncomfortable to bitch about such high-quality, first-world problems, especially when conceiving at all is such a blessing.

Later, when I end up talking about the pregnancy publicly, and all the symptoms that go along with it, I get an angry e-mail: "I used to be a fan of yours, but my husband and I can't conceive and I am sick of hearing you complain about being pregnant."

She has a point and now my worst fears about how I'm coming across are confirmed. That's when I ask myself, who *can* complain? My girlfriend who is desperate to get married and pushing forty-five up a hill would probably be pissed off at this bitch for bemoaning the fact that she can't conceive when at least she is lucky enough to have found a mate. Someone else would hate the forty-five-year-old for griping because at least she has a job, even if she hasn't found a man. Take this thesis to its natural end and there is one guy living under a bridge with no arms, no job, no parents and maybe one kidney who has the right to complain. And only that guy. So the argument is spurious and I'll continue to lament all I goddamn want.

Back to complaining, although I promise to try and keep it in perspective and tritely struggle to find the bright side, because that makes me feel better about complaining the way knocking wood makes me feel better about having hope.

My biggest complaint in these early days, and it's one that will grow and fester, is anxiety, which is alleviated only by my doctor visits every couple of weeks. My doctor is one of these guys who gives you an ultrasound every time you go to the office, probably because he bought the expensive imaging machine and insurance covers the test so patients don't sweat it and it doesn't hurt and everyone loves to see their fetus on-screen and ascribe all kinds of bullshit characteristics to it, so why not blast sound waves at your fetus unnecessarily? Anyway, at my eight-week checkup, I sit on the butcher paper during my exam as he probes me with the transducer, my denim skirt in a pile with my panties in the corner, my husband in the other corner, and there it is: the heartbeat. He turns up the volume and we can hear it, fast and loud, calling us to the other side.

Now I think I can talk about the baby, but I'm not sure.

I take the small black-and-white photo from the ultrasound like I'm going to be all scrapbookish, but it ends up stuffed in my glove compartment.

In a way, this is sad. In another way, it's reassuring. My therapist was right—maybe I'll still just be me, but with a kid. I will not suddenly turn into, say, this woman whose pregnancy blog I found online complete with a photo of herself in jeans and an unbuttoned white shirt. In the picture, her husband stands behind her, also in jeans and a white shirt, and both of them make heart shapes with their hands surrounding her belly button. Even if you don't have morning sickness, this will probably make you throw up in your mouth. At least I know I can find less syrupy ways of disgusting people with my solipsism. Or at least I fundamentally understand that despite the thrill of being "a little bit pregnant," a sonogram image of my fetus at eight weeks is not compelling to anyone else. Like the dried-out ballpoint pen, melted ChapStick and expired insurance cards also rattling around in my glove box, its usefulness has passed.

The likelihood of miscarrying seems smaller now that I've seen the fetus, and I'm increasingly anxious to tell. Mostly, I want to tell the listeners of the radio show, who have been with me through Billy, the guy who met the love of his life when I declared us "on a three-month break"; Anton, the guy I met on MySpace and almost married in Vegas on our first date before I sobered up; and countless other dating misadventures, not to mention the blaring sound of a clock ticking that our sound effects guy, Bald Bryan, had been playing for years whenever I discussed my personal life. The morning show is going off the air, because the station is flipping from talk to Top 40. After almost three years, I just want this one moment with the anonymous masses who have traveled with me. I want it though it isn't prudent; I want to tell though I know there is no way to un-tell a couple of million people, what with the show going off the air and all. I would wait the entire twelve weeks, but I can't because the end is nigh and 97.1 FM will not be a place for anecdotes, but instead for a steady dose of Taylor Swift and Lady Gaga.

Our last day is a Friday, a month before I'm officially out of pregatory. I still have no idea whether I'm going to say anything on the air. As always, Adam Carolla throws it to me to do the news. I hear my news music through my headphones (or "cans," as I like to say to act like I know what I'm doing) and I have no idea what I'm going to do. There is a pause while I grip a stack of the day's news in my sweaty hands.

"The lead story today . . . I'm pregnant."

Adam is so touched, he has his assistant Jay run into the studio and hug me.

I get my dramatic moment, lots of callers congratulating me, and coworkers running in to squeeze me and mistake my estrogen surge for a "glow."

Though I've now spilled the beans to a couple million listeners, I don't call my mom. I sometimes think she will call me, when she hears it through the grapevine or reads it online, but I know that comes from the fantasy place of the little girl who thinks her mom will do lots of things she won't—pick her up from school when it's raining, smile at her when she enters a room, tape her lousy drawings to the refrigerator, be able to name her elementary school teacher.

Now, if my uterus plays its cards right, I'm going to be someone's mom, and the only good thing about this rising level of concern for my baby is that it proves I'm already attached. My constant worry is like a friend whispering in my ear, or perhaps posting a note on my esophagus written in stomach acid and bile, saying, "You will not be your mother." You will fuck it up in your own way, but not in hers.

five

I'll Miss You, Toxins

Even someone like me who isn't particularly good with babies, who looks at them and says things like, "Hey, buddy. Look at your little face," before resorting to a flaccid round of peek-a-boo and then running out of material, even I endeavor to err on the side of caution when it comes to chemicals. After years of wondering if I'm cut out to be a mother, I'm relieved to find that the instinct to protect this fetus is so strong, or at least the image of me smoking a Camel while balancing a tumbler of Jameson on my bulging stomach is so distasteful, that I figure all of my favorite chemicals can wait.

And I really love chemicals.

Being pregnant makes me feel toward booze and Xanax and Retin-A the way Emily from *Our Town* felt about food, hot baths and milk delivered to your door. She didn't appreciate the simple things in life until she returned as a ghost to Grover's Corners, relived one day as her twelve-year-old self, and asked the question all preteen girls agonize over while performing Emily's big monologue at theater camp: "Does anyone ever realize life while they live it?"

What I mean is, I never appreciated guilt-free drug use until it was gone. Did I just compare not using Klonopin to dying? Is that overblown? Someone get me to Samuel French because I'm feeling dramatic.

I had no idea how much I took the privilege of occasionally poisoning myself for granted until now. I've always been moderate about my use of prescription drugs and alcohol, yet my pregnant longing for a lightly altered state makes me feel (and come across) like a flat-out junkie. No matter. The fact is this: I'm pregnant, which means I've got way more worries than ever before, and way fewer chemicals to make them go away.

Chemicals, I can't wait to return to you. Until then, here is a list of the substances I miss the most.

VICODIN—Narcotics are bad. Except for the fact they produce a little something called euphoria. Listen, this drug is a highly addictive opioid that should be used only to manage moderate to severe pain. However, my definition of "pain" is a loose one. Is it painful to sit around pondering labor, the mysterious process of somehow squeezing a human head out of your va-jay-jay? Does it smart to look down the pike at childbirth, something most of us have only seen in movies (during which the woman sweats profusely, swears, wails, curses her husband and, let's face it, dies half the time)? Speaking of death, does it hurt emotionally to ponder the absolute *end* of one's identity? Is it a bit of an *ouchy* to imagine never going to the gym, the nail salon, or the therapist, without first scheduling a sitter? Does it ache to even hear yourself say the word "sitter"? If a future of pureeing yams to make your own baby food causes a throbbing in your very terrified soul, well, you are in moderate to severe pain. When painkillers are prescribed "as needed," I always feel "as needed" is a very fluid concept. Medicines are categorized in various ways as it pertains to their use during pregnancy. The FDA says Vicodin is a category C drug, meaning it is unknown whether it would be harmful to an unborn baby. Since there haven't been adequate or well-controlled studies, since vitamin V is habit-forming and may depress the baby's breathing if taken late in the third trimester, most doctors won't sign off on this and neither will your conscience.

Incidentally, any drug worth your time will probably be a category C, which should stand for "Could be fine but you'll feel like a selfish baby maimer if it's not." Category B drugs are considered "probably safe," and include such party favorites as Tylenol and Pepcid. We've all heard about those underground Pep/Ty raves. All the kids are rolling on P and T, saying *Screw E, we're up in here with mild relief of muscle aches and almost no heartburn. Join us in this unfettered pleasure-fest. It's a pharmaceutical bacchanal.* Even though Vicodin means I'm twenty minutes from the sense that all is right with the world, I'm off the junk.

KLONOPIN—Relaxes muscles, reduces anxiety, helps you sleep, features a nice long half-life so you wake up fresh as a daisy and worry-free. Take it the night before a job interview or audition and the entire next day is kissed with a light potion of placidity. Klony seemed so harmless until I read that when taken during pregnancy it may cause "floppy infant syndrome." I don't know what that is, and I don't want to know.

NICOTINE—C'mon. Smoking sucks. I get it. But how else are you supposed to know when dinner is over?

Of all of my darling toxins, I'm shocked to miss smoking the most. Nicotine was never and is not now a physical addiction for me (I'm what's known as a "chipper," someone who smokes a few cigarettes regularly but never becomes a pack-a-day smoker). I know nicotine is bad. I quit smoking my two to three after-dinner puffy treats as soon as I realized I was pregnant. Though we went way back together, I was never John Wayne with the smokes, and I always thought letting go of one or two cigarettes would be easy. I wasn't a real smoker, never even smoked during daylight hours.

Right now, I don't want to smoke just a couple.

I want to sit in bed and chain-smoke while high on half a Vicodin and watch a couple of documentaries like I used to do on a Friday night when the mood struck. Smoking calms nerves, and I've never been more nervous than I am about this baby: how he's doing in there, how he is going to get out, when I'm going to ascertain the meaning of the word "layette" or make myself care about the best brand of disposable nipple pads.

It's hard to talk about smoking without pissing people off. Folks get way more irate about smoking than if I happened to orchestrate dog fights, because their uncle died a horrible death of lung cancer or their brother burned down an apartment building because he was smoking in bed or they're allergic to smoke and have had an ashtray full of sitting next to rude butt suckers blithely contaminating their fresh air. I'm sorry. I'm so, so sorry. You people are right. There is no defending smoking; there is just the truth for me. There were nights writing on deadline when smokes were my editor and my roommate, solo road trips during which cigs were my passenger, helping me stay alert through the desert, stay brave at stranded rest stops. Smokes have been my date to parties, my therapist after breakups, my diet aid and my inspirational carrot, dangling ahead of me as a reward for anything from finishing an article to getting through a family reunion.

Each time I quiet the flirtatious come-on of a Camel Light, it's comforting to know my early maternal instincts outweigh the brute force of habit and several bassinets full of anxiety.

Seems like this would be a great opportunity to just quit for good. Instead I wish I could first have a baby and then immediately have a cigarette in the recovery room.

XANAX—Oh, yummy Xanax, first given to me by a makeup artist before I had to spend three hours on a freezing cold red carpet interviewing more important people on their way into a party celebrating the one thousandth episode of a late-night show, they make things easier.

I usually quarter these pills, never take the whole thing, though I often try to mix with one cocktail for maximum buzz (when the label reads "this medication may increase the effects of alcohol," I take that as a helpful hint).

Xanax is not my go-to pill. Admired by anxious pill poppers for its ability to act quickly, it has a short half-life in your body. This is useful if you are having an unscheduled meltdown, but the tranquility is short-lived. There are usually a few of these rolling around in my shoebox full of "dolls," but I rarely use them, maybe three times a year. Panic attacks aren't my thing as much as cultivating a constant, low level of dread. Still, I miss the option. If my heart starts pounding and my stomach starts churning and I suddenly can't stop my mind from racing, I'm walking a terror tightrope with no chemical net.

Sure, there are side effects. Oh, no! I might be afflicted with drowsiness, lightheadedness, euphoria and disinhibition! Wait. I desperately want those things.

ARTIFICIAL SWEETENERS—Yellow packets, blue packets, pink, I don't know what's in you or which of you is better, but you all taste so chemical-y now. You taste like a birth defect. Half a Splenda in my beverage is my sweetener threshold before the fear and guilt set in, and that's a far cry from the three packs I used to enjoy in my cereal just for the fuck of it.

BOOZE—Nursing is about to mean something totally different, I know, but it used to be what I did to two fingers of room-temp single malt Scotch. What rounds out the edges now? Anyone who suggests a hot bath or meditating or chamomile tea is going to get punched in the face.

I know. I should process all my fears by reaching out, or by "sitting with the feelings." If the feelings are sitting on a bar stool, I'll sit with them and have a nice full-bodied pinot. Otherwise, I don't like sitting with my feelings. It's like sitting with an obese teenager on a cross-country flight, uncomfortable and sad.

My doctor didn't sweat me having one or two last cigarettes before my sixth week. Though he didn't love it, he could see the need for gradual weaning. That being said, he is categorically against drinking alcohol in pregnancy. His hard-line attitude about Drinking While Gestating is sobering. Literally.

The man said I could smoke, something society sees as tantamount to bunny drowning, but allows not one drop of liquor. My pregnant friends, they are all wink-wink about a nightly half glass of wine, and most doctors say a very moderate amount of booze in the third trimester is fine, but my doctor's warning haunts me.

At a restaurant in Napa, the sommelier gives us one of these: "My mom drank when she was pregnant with me and I'm fine." You hear that a lot, and anyone who says that to you is probably a good person and should be befriended or tipped well. It's true, in the course of modern human history, lots of moms drank and most of those babies are fine, like Betty Draper's kids are fine, like mine will probably be fine if I decide to take my medical advice from a sommelier.

Giving up alcohol is relatively easy for me, so I basically do it. Like getting dumped by a guy you never really liked, you get lots of sympathy, but inside, you aren't exactly crushed.

Experts are all over the place with this one, so take what I'm saying with a grain of salt, which is the only thing left you *can* take.

ADVIL—I never used this much, but now that I can't, I realize it was nice to have around. Headache, pain, inflammation? Live with it, because you probably shouldn't pop anything containing ibuprofen. They say watermelon helps reduce inflammation, and I'm shoving some down my gullet daily to address the puffiness that has overtaken me, but really, ingesting some cubes of fruit to do what a pill should be doing? That hippie nonsense is right up there with warm milk to help you sleep and petting a puppy to reduce blood pressure. Bogus.

CAFFEINE—I have a decaf now and again, but some scary article I read when I was trying to get pregnant linked excessive coffee drinking with an increased rate of miscarriage. As losing this baby is the stickiest, most pernicious worry I've ever had, it seems like every caffeinated beverage is just a miscarriage-a-ccino.

Green tea, diet soft drinks, chocolate, *no más*. I know I'm not downing a thalidomide milk shake with a DES chaser, but my guiding principle is starting to be when in doubt, leave it out.

With coffee, it's not so much the buzz I miss as the experience, the ritual, the palming of the overpriced latte, the constant refills of diner coffee at breakfast, the sight of my environmentally friendly plastic mug in my car's cup holder. I've never trusted people who don't drink coffee because "yuck, it tastes bitter" or "eeew, it makes me wired." Wired and bitter are defining qualities that I now have to give up to make room for some kind of earth mother, mellow, natural vibe that just may never come, well, naturally.

RETIN-A—Careful, constant and expensive grooming helps me address the genetic hand I was dealt, not a total bust but a pair of threes at best. With a few bucks and some toxic treatments, I can look all right. Now, I'm pregnant and won't even have that saving grace of chubby women everywhere, a pretty face.

Who knows if it works, but they say Retin-A staves off breakouts and wrinkles and I have both right now as my prescription tube sits in the drawer, expiring. Oh, goody, now I can buy organic lotions with powerful ingredients like sunflower seed oil, witch hazel and willow bark extract. Great. My dermatologist reminds me that I can start using it again after the baby is born . . . oh, wait, no, after I'm done breast-feeding, so in, like, a million years. Likewise, Botox is out and so is any other skin treatment that is remotely effective. Salicylic acid, which is in most of the random lotions I keep around to slap on breakouts, is also out. I'm not supposed to be concerned about anything as silly as the condition of my skin now that I'm creating new life, but I'm not creating a new personality free of self-consciousness, and I'm also not creating a world free of reflective surfaces. Now I have two chins, and both are breaking out.

HAIR COLOR—Some say it's okay to use, others say just get highlights and don't let the noxious formula touch your scalp, but let's face it, who wants to sit in the salon all pregnant while women judge you for caring more about your roots than your baby? Hairdresser to me: "What do you think these giant smocks are for? Hiding the belly. Pleeeeaaase. I work on pregnant women every day." And hairdressers with this attitude, should, of course, be kept close to your heart. However, if I'm choosing toxins like it's Sophie's Choice, this one doesn't make it.

SELF-TANNER—Again, lots of pregnant girls use it and it's probably fine. If you search long enough, you'll find some Dr. Buzzkill to dissuade you from most delicious chemicals, as does ob-gyn Suzanne Gilberg-Lenz, who writes, "I tell my patients to avoid chemical tanning at the very least in the first trimester, when the majority of fetal organ formation occurs." Ha, lady! I'll wait for the second trimester.

Not so fast. She adds that brain development continues throughout pregnancy and that skin is the largest organ in the body, thus making it more dangerous to expose it to the active ingredient in tanners, DHA (dihydroxyacetone). Fine. *Fine.* If there is a better way to gloss over the aesthetic challenges of being both pregnant and just generally over thirty, I haven't found it. DHA, IOU. And I miss you.

EveryGoddamnThing—involves chemicals. Your moisturizer is suspect, your soap seems to have a long list of ingredients with too many consonants. Your eye cream smells too good and doesn't go bad for too long to be trusted. Your nail polish seems like a close cousin to lead paint. The fumes at the gas station are out to get you, as is the air when you roll down your window on the freeway, and even your laundry detergent seems like venom. The entire world suddenly seems artificially colored and flavored and threatening to tamper with your fragile, defenseless fetus.

I am going to drop a heavy name. Tori Spelling. That's right. I interview her and her second husband for my show on deep cable. She's recently birthed her second baby and is beautifully exploiting it with both a reality show and a book. Because I'm pregnant, we have a girl chat off-camera during which I confide my desire for just one Ambien to help me sleep.

Mind you, Tori and I have a lot in common. Both of us have trouble with our unforgiving, chilly mothers. Of course, hers forced her to get a nose job and mine forced me to get a *job* job, but we're basically the same person. Okay, her dad produced *The Love Boat* and my dad, California's only Jewish auto mechanic, has produced nothing but years of rebuilt alternators and debt more toxic than an asbestos onesie, but now that I'm with child, there is a bridge between me and anyone else who has ever been here. We cover our microphones and Tori whispers that her doctor said hair color was fine, same with the occasional Ambien, and I know deep inside myself that I have made my last Tori Spelling joke. Bless her.

Half an Ambien gets me through one sleepless night, but I go back to abstaining. Briefly, I consider the herbal sleep remedy, melatonin, but guess what? A quick Google search confirms my fear: It's not recommended during pregnancy. That's right, now you can't even put your bench-warming sleep aids in the game.

Funny thing, though. The more hushed conversations or e-mail exchanges I have with moms, the more I start to formulate a theory about pregnancy and toxins: *Everyone lies.* Maybe not with their first babies, because we first-timers are all trepidatious and terrified, but once they get to that second, third, fourth pregnancy, *they lie.* They use moderation and common sense, and they keep their minimal toxic exposures under their hats, with their dyed hair.

I'm still a rookie, though, and I don't have the balls. The avoidance of chemicals for me is mostly about the avoidance of future guilt. If this kid has even a skosh of floppy baby syndrome, how will I know it wasn't the result of three minutes in the Mystic Tan booth? I'm better safe than sorry; it's just that safe doesn't win by much.

People I Want to Punch: Bummer Ladies

I f one more mom tells me, "Go to the movies now, because after you have the baby you'll never get to go to the movies again," or "Go on a trip now, because once you have the baby you'll never leave town again," or "Have a date night now, because you will never see your husband again," I am going to punch her right in her tired, defeated face.

Hey, how about you shut your rude, projecting, bitter soup coolers and let me be?

Just let me deal with the fact that I feel like I've been strapped to the spinning teacup ride at goddamn Dizzyland for the last fifteen weeks.

Allow my nauseated, terrified, pregnancy-hobbled brain to stick to its usual troubling fare, and by that I mean nonstop oscillating between thoughts of various fatal genetic defects and how best to phrase it to people if I end up having a "nonviable pregnancy."

Stop to consider that as a first-time mom-to-be, I'm kind of overstocked with worries right now. It's like you're peddling mortgage-backed securities to AIG. *No gracias*, I got enough of those and they're all toxic, anyway.

To see me all bulging about the middle is to know I'm already in too deep, so keep it to yourself if you think my life will be a dingy wasteland once my bundle of joy-lessness arrives.

Let's talk about a girl named Kim.

Having heard I was pregnant, she messaged me on Facebook with the following advice: "Take a look at your body right now, because it will never look this way again. Your stomach will be so pockmarked and stretched out, there will be nothing you can do about it, so enjoy it now."

I barely know this woman, and while I am impressed at her ability to paint such a richly hued portrait of how crappy I'm going to look, I can't understand what drives her other than pure evil.

Susceptibility to stretch marks is genetic, and they may also be exacerbated by excessive or rapid weight gain. However, what if there is another, more mysteri-ous cause? What if the collagen gods punish people like Kim for being passive-aggressive twats?

You can't laser that away, Kimmy. See you on Punch You in the Facebook.

If I do morph into a bleary-eyed, pockmarked, sad sack with spit-up and organic oatmeal in my hair who is too neurotically attached to her precious child to allow anyone to babysit, I hope to have enough compassion to lie my saggy ass off when I see a pregnant girl and simply say, "You are going to love being a mom."

six

CVS: Order Now and Enjoy Six Months (Worry) Free!

I don't want to say I get the hard sell on having a CVS test, but when I go to my mandatory pretest genetic counseling session, it feels a little like being on a used car lot on the last day of the month taking a recession test drive with a salesman one vehicle short of his quota.

The facts: The CVS (chorionic villus sampling) is often offered to women who will be over thirty-five on their due date, who have a family history of certain birth defects or who tested positive for genetic disorders. I will be thirty-nine on my due date, and am a carrier for both Tay-Sachs disease and cystic fibrosis, so I qualify for the procedure, which involves removing some cells from the placenta for diagnostic testing. It's similar to an amniocentesis, but can be done earlier, between ten and thirteen weeks. There are risks involved, namely miscarriage, which some sources say occurs in one out of every hundred procedures. On the other hand, the statistics are murky, because miscarriage rates are higher during these weeks anyway, and in the hands of a skilled practitioner the risks may be lower.

Amniocentesis is also supposedly risky, but it's almost impossible for me to gauge the exact numbers, so I Google myself into a tizzy and end up sitting in the geneticist's office jumping through all of the hospital's hoops so I can leave my options open before the window of opportunity slams shut on the CVS for good.

We review our family histories, the usual cancer and heart disease type stuff, before the counselor breaks out the *Big Book of Genetic Disorders*, which he flips through to show us what we might be facing blindly should we forgo the CVS, scheduled for the following morning.

For almost every chromosome, there is some possible abnormality.

In essence, as he pushes the book toward us, he's asking, "What's it going to take to get you into these stirrups?" And he isn't going to let us walk without closing.

I'm sure the information is medically sound, responsible, factual, but this is pretty much how I hear it.

Mrs. Strasser, this CVS is top of the line. It's the Cadillac of invasive prenatal diagnostic tests, and we give you a lifetime no chromosomal defects guarantee!

Now, if you like "uncertainty," perhaps this test isn't for you. I guess you don't mind the idea of visiting your child in an institution because it's severely impaired and you just didn't feel like getting the CVS. I guess you are one of those people who don't mind Fragile X syndrome or spinal muscular atrophy. Look, the CVS test is not for everyone, just customers who appreciate our 99 percent accuracy rate in diagnosing chromosomal abnormalities.

We offer easy financing through your insurance company.

But really, how can you put a price on peace of mind? Our model CVS practitioner, Dr. Everyone Goes to Him, is the best on the market. Best safety record around. On the other hand, like I said, some folks don't care about safety, and if that's you, I guess the CVS isn't an investment worth making right now.

Let me show you some of the other CVS features.

We can test for several hundred genetic disorders. You carry Tay-Sachs disease? Cystic fibrosis? We got you covered. Did you say you were Ashkenazi? Yikes, that's bad. What? Nothing.

The first trimester screening test you already had, that nice little sonogram and blood screen combo, that's cute and all, but if you want a real test, that's a waste of your time. Sure, that checks for a few mutations, but this is the bad boy. We check all twenty-three chromosomes. Order now, and we'll even throw in free gender identification.

You can think about it, but at twelve weeks, you don't have much time. Dr. Everyone Goes to Him books up and your window for this test closes at thirteen weeks. No pressure. You can have an amniocentesis at fifteen weeks if you like. Up to you. But I sure wouldn't want to run into any defects that late in the game.

Sold.

My husband is against it. He feels confident that, based on the noninvasive screening we already had, the baby is fine, that the risks aren't worth it.

Sure, even if one in a hundred of these things causes a miscarriage, we still have a 99 percent chance of coming out fine, which sounds so promising when you look at it that way, like an A+ grade, unless you are that one in a hundred, in which case you get an F, for Fucked.

I am up all night making lists, weighing pros and cons like I did before we conceived. If this test harms the baby, I won't be able to live with myself, but if the baby has problems, I want to know about it. Moreover, I want to rest assured. I never rest, and I'm rarely assured, but maybe this will help set my mind at ease. I just don't know about six months of not knowing for certain; I don't think I can hack it. It's the most difficult decision I've ever made and I wonder if parenting is just going to be more of the same: high-stakes choices that make you wish for gut instincts, but leave you with only the conflicting advice of experts.

With just enough time to get there and park, I decide to go for it.

When we arrive, there is a preliminary ultrasound. I've always known it's a girl, and now I'm positive, because of her pretty fetal cheekbones and my newfound mommy juju. They can't tell until they look at the placenta cells, but I know. Now I just have to get through this test, to make sure she's okay. My husband and I wait for the doctor, who breezes in, distracted, looking at his watch.

"Um, good morning. I might need to step out. Got a nonviable pregnancy next door. Waiting to hear from their doctor," he says, looking down at a chart.

I don't want the guy scooping my ice cream cone to be distracted, because he might give me an undersize portion, or place it on the cone insecurely. But the guy who is about to stick a needle in my placenta? I would really like him to be totally focused.

What's more, as my legs get cold and purple in the stirrups, it dawns on me that "nonviable fetus" is a nice way of saying dead baby. *Dead baby.* That nice couple we saw in the waiting room, the guy with shaggy hair under a baseball cap and the lady in a long brown sweater nibbling on crackers, their day started just like ours, only their routine ultrasound ended up revealing a dead baby, nonviable as a doornail, which now needs to be removed by their ob-gyn, who can't be located. I imagine them huddled under fluorescent lights, trying to process this hideous turn of events, just on the other side of the wall, just a few yards away from us.

I'm filled with pregnancy-hormone-soaked grief for these strangers, and the thought of them stops me nonviable in my tracks.

"Do we start now or wait until this thing gets resolved? You know what? Let's just do it. Let's make hay while the sun shines," the doctor announces, and a few nurses snap into action. "Knock if their OB calls," he yells out to the receptionist.

Dead baby!!!

Next thing you know, he's inserting a needle into my body to biopsy the placental tissue and making small talk.

"Where are you from? San Francisco? Do you know the biggest city in the Bay Area?"

Let me think. Dead baby? No, that can't be right.

"Oakland?" I croak, trying to show how casual I am, how easygoing.

"Relax. The worst thing you can do is tense up. The only thing that can go wrong is if you're not relaxed, you move a little, the muscles tense up in there and I can't get the needle in, so I really need you to relax. I do a lot of these, and the only problems I run into are from women who tighten up," he warns.

Can't be one of these "tighten up" types, women who ruin it and kill their babies because they can't settle down.

That's when I will myself into stillness, attempt a mind-over-matter swami thing where I clear my mind and force my body into a state of calm.

"San Jose," he says. "Can you believe it?"

Usually, I couldn't care less about geography, or whether I'm good at trivia, don't mind intentionally throwing party games like Celebrity so we can all be done and play an even better game called Drinking and Conversing, but I'm intensely bothered that I guessed Oakland.

The doctor is black. Oakland has a large black population, and I start thinking that he thinks I guessed Oakland because I'm racist and was just thinking black because of my black doctor and I start getting paranoid that he is going to dislike my Oakland-guessing ass and unconsciously play fast and loose with the placenta poking. This delusional level of discourse is calling the shots in my frontal cortex, but still I relax my pelvic muscles.

Dead baby, my brain tries to shout, but gets muzzled by the swami.

He gets what he needs without incident. In seconds, he's out the door and I'm instructed to get my clothes on and everyone is going about their business wrapping up when I realize I can't move. Something is very wrong. I'm clammy and faint. I don't want to alarm my husband, but I'm so hot all I can think about is getting to the bathroom floor, where I can sprawl out like a dog and cool down my body temperature. I need to throw up. My shoes, skirt and panties are across the room and I calculate correctly that I really need only the skirt, which I pull on and attempt a nonchalant jaunt to the bathroom.

On the cool linoleum of the bathroom floor, I apologize to god for making such a huge mistake. I make lots of deals about the saintly way I'm going to live if god lets me keep this baby. I'm not very religious. I just use the word "god" as shorthand for the universe, or a power greater than myself, or the force, or whatever thing I pray to when I've just run out of options and figure it can't hurt. Daniel will never forgive me for doing this, I tell god. I just couldn't leave well enough alone and I am so sorry. However conflicted I may have been about procreating, I want this baby.

I start to cool down. Not because of divine intervention, probably, but just my blood pressure normalizing.

Forcing myself to get up because I know my husband must be panicking by now, I stumble back toward the room, where a couple of nurses tell me I am looking green. "It's not easy being green," I reply, because you don't come up with your best material when you've just been on a germy floor making deals and choking down vomit.

My blood pressure has plummeted. The nurses give me some juice and instruct me to get back on the table. The doctor is called. He rushes in and takes another look at my insides via ultrasound and informs me that I am having a uterine contraction, points it out on the screen, explains something about my vagus nerve flooding my body with adrenaline, which caused the contraction. Apparently, this isn't an uncommon response to stress; the body sometimes maintains equilibrium until the threat passes, after which it's safe to spaz out.

"Everything is fine. The procedure went perfectly," he says.

"Why isn't the baby moving?" I ask, craning my head to stare at the sonogram screen.

"It's asleep."

"Can you wake it up?"

He jostles my stomach. Jostles it pretty hard. The kid won't budge.

"That's okay. As long as you swear the baby is fine."

"It's fine."

They send me home with instructions to stay flat for twenty-four hours, just get up to pee and that's it. We pay extra to get the results sooner, and when the lab finally phones, I miss the call, but I recognize the number and my vagus nerve starts doing its thing again as I retrieve the voice mail.

"This is Jen from the lab. The news is good. Give me a call."

I know leaving these messages is a delicate task and I don't know this Jen, but I want to hug her and fill out some kind of comment card about what a great job she is doing, what a perfect tone she strikes. When I get her on the line, she simply says, "Everything is normal. Do you want to know the gender?"

Of course I do, because I really just want to confirm that I'm getting my girl, the one we are going to name Harper, after Harper Lee. My world is transformed. I know my baby is healthy and I know she is a girl, and that I'm going to give her cute Suri Cruise bangs and that we're going to paint the town pink together and that I won't force her to take ballet, but that she'll probably insist on wearing her princess outfit to the supermarket, where the butcher will remark on her gorgeous eyes and give her a lollipop. A pink lollipop.

"It's a boy."

People I Want to Punch: Just Grateful for a Healthy Baby

There are two kinds of people who tell you they don't have a gender preference when it comes to their baby: big fat liars, and women so well adjusted that they aren't counting on their kid to help them resolve any issues from their childhood. I don't know which category I want to punch more.

If you're lying, I understand that you want to appear angelic and gracious, but your lies do a disservice to humanity. Okay, maybe that's overstating it, but your fakery makes those of us with a preference feel alone and possibly makes us doubt our readiness to even be mothers at all. So, shame on you for fronting. And shame on me for using that term and trying to front that I'm so gangsta.

Maybe you are lying to yourself, and have convinced yourself you don't care about gender. Or maybe you are knowingly fibbing so people won't judge you. You know what? Lying is kind of a garden-variety sin and I'm not that mad at you.

Now, to those of you who truly don't care, I have a delicious knuckle sandwich with your name on it. Since you're pregnant, I might as well stuff it with unpasteurized cheese and mercury-laden fish.

Because you are fine with either gender, you do some really mystifying things, like ask your doctor and ultrasound technicians to keep it a secret from you. You make a big to-do about how excited you are to find out when the baby is born, like it's going to add to the orgy of organic glee and maternal righteousness that will be your birth experience, like you and your family will have a delightful surprise awaiting you at the end of your vaginal canal, while we gender-finder-outers will be digging into the bottom of a box of Cracker Jack to find no prize, just a handful of boring old crumbs.

When you discuss the Big Reveal that's coming your way, it's as though you really know how to live, how to embrace the mysteries of existence, how to make every rite of passage a theme party thrown by a socialite in the Hamptons. Meanwhile, the rest of us will be wearing wilted party hats and drinking sparkling cider at the retirement party of a middle-management drone named Phyllis.

A hallmark of your ilk is that you are known to use the insidious phrase "We don't care if it's a boy or a girl; we just want a healthy baby." Which is another way of saying that we who prefer one gender to the other *don't care at all* about our baby's well-being, as long as we can paint the nursery blue or pink and make our own narcissistic dreams come true.

If you are pregnant, the number-one question you get asked is this: "Are you having a boy or a girl?" If you don't care, you get to pull out the "healthy baby" chestnut, and even though it kind of grinds the conversation to a halt, it really is the way to go.

In my case, I answer "Boy" with a forlorn look and brief explanation about how I'm not that thrilled about years of toy cars and gas jokes, or barely cute little-boy outfits like mini cargo pants and stupid "Daddy's Team" T-shirts. I have to try to keep it light, though, so I can still tell the truth while not conveying the real disappointment that makes me kind of a crappy person and dangerously close to revisiting the mean-spiritedness of my own mom with her "It's a Boy" cards. I have to button it with something positive, like "Boys love their mommies!"

You who are buying yellow and white baby swings and onesies, who *just want a healthy baby*, I salute you. You are superior. However, don't be surprised if on my way to saluting you, my hand gets confused, balls into a fist, and lands in your face.

seven

Bad Move: Calling Nancy O'Dell
a Stupid C-Word

Almost every idiotic thing I do can be traced back to one basic flaw: trying too hard. This explains how I end up calling Nancy O'Dell a "stupid c-word."

Her publicist sends me a copy of O'Dell's book, *Full of Life: Mom-to-Mom Tips I Wish Someone Had Told Me When I Was Pregnant*, and I settle down to read it one afternoon after work, Cherry Mylanta by my side, clutter I'm too tired to clean crowding our tiny condo. This is just what I need today, I figure, some insider information from Nancy O'Dell, the former host of *Access Hollywood* and a onetime Miss South Carolina. She's going to tell me things she wishes she had known, maybe provide a bit of commiseration.

Of course, you can't have "commiserate" without its Latin root, "miser," which means "wretched," and Nancy doesn't experience much wretchedness, mostly just glee expressed with an abundance of unironic exclamation points. I sip a bit of antacid while reading about her absence of pregnancy nausea. My morning sickness increases just reading about her lack of it. While I hope my ponytail is long enough to cover up the cystic acne on the back of my neck, I read about Nancy's pregnancy skin.

"I swear it actually glowed. It was luminous and smooth. Now, you have to understand, every day I sit in a chair for over an hour while makeup is applied to my skin to create that *very same glow!*"

Jealousy grips me as I grip her book in my sweaty hands and I continue reading about her awesome skin.

"I'd read that an increase in hormones could sometimes cause the opposite reaction, aggravating skin and causing breakouts. Phew, I had dodged a bullet there!" writes Nancy. And guess what? That bullet she dodged hit me right in the face, and anywhere else one might find a sebaceous gland.

There wasn't going to be much commiserating, but maybe I could get something out of those mom-to-mom tips.

"I recommend that you start your baby scrapbook on the day of your first ultrasound, the first time you see your little one. Granted, it may just look like a dot on the page, but that's your baby!" She includes a handy chart of other things to include in your scrapbook, including "close-ups of nursery furniture and bedding" and "nursery paint color samples." I'm not sure where I'm even going to fit a crib, and I'm also not sure if that first ultrasound photo is still in my glove compartment, or if I tossed it out with some unpaid parking tickets and take-out menus.

Moving on, I check out some of her wardrobe tips.

Drawstring pants are very useful, she reveals, adding that you can hide your belly with a long scarf. "A large designer bag will do the trick as well, so this gives you a good excuse to buy one!"

Neat. Thanks for that mom-to-mom tip everyone can use; everyone, that is, with a couple thousand bucks to spend on a Gucci satchel.

She and her husband both felt in their hearts they were having a girl, but naturally, they would have been happy either way. Well, their hearts were right, and her CVS test confirmed that baby girl Ashby was on her way.

It wasn't all hearts and flowers. She was "forgetful" and often had to have her husband scratch her itchy belly with a towel, but even that process was "Heaven, I tell you. Better than any cream. And better than doing it yourself!"

Nancy also battled constipation, leg cramps and dizziness, but all of those problems had easy solutions: Stay hydrated, make your mom's famous spice cake recipe with extra prunes and "put your feet up as much as possible."

Paging through her trimesters, I discover she does have one real difficulty. The matching ottoman, glider, changing table and crib for Ashby will take eight to ten weeks to be delivered, not making it in time for the baby's arrival, and the material for the nursery curtains is on back order as well. To make matters worse, her second choice of curtain fabric has been discontinued! "So place your orders with enough time to allow for delays." Noted. I'll make sure to let my decorator know.

Finally, I get to the best part. Nancy is holding her baby, and she's in tears. Tears. Now we're getting somewhere.

She just can't understand why she's crying when having a baby was so richly rewarding. That's when her husband diagnoses her with her single, serious baby-related disorder.

"Babe, what you have is *postpartum elation.*"

I groan and toss the book under the coffee table with a pile of other books never to be read again. Nancy is now out of sight, but not out of mind. The more I think about her, the more I resent this perky, blonde stranger (now selling her own jewelry line on QVC).

When it's time to sit in with Adam Carolla to record his podcast the next day, I'm still thinking about America's sweetheart and the tiny white crochet booties with lavender ribbons on the cover of her book, and her whole blessing-filled pregnancy, especially as I discuss mine, a stark contrast. Full of life, but also full of fear, self-doubt and acne.

I guess I got caught up in the moment, trying to be funny, trying to fit in with Adam and the guys at the studio, trying to be so bracingly honest that pregnant women everywhere would embrace me as their new truth teller and anti-O'Dell.

Let's face it, after three years of not cursing on FM radio I was a little "fuck" and "asshole" happy, but there was no need to go "c-word" on Nancy and I was way, way out of line, trying to make a point and, as is always the case when I am trying too hard, saying something lame.

After recording the podcast, I wake up in a panic in the middle of the night, "full" of regret. Nancy O'Dell will probably never even hear the show, I realize, and wouldn't care if she did, because she has a life (is, as I've noted, *Full of Life*), but it doesn't matter, because I know I said it and it came out all wrong, as only the c-word can.

Nancy, if you happen to read this, I am so sorry.

I know you can't relate, because according to your book your worst pregnancy symptom was frightfully lustrous hair, but I'm kind of unhinged right now.

You couldn't stop crying because having a daughter (Ashby!) made you think of your own beloved mother and the goddamn circle of goddamn life. Meanwhile, I lost the mom lottery and haven't even spoken to my own mother this entire pregnancy, a pain that you poked with your literary outpouring of family joy. In every fundamental way that you had and are a mother, I got nothing.

Whereas, Nancy, you are perfect. You have everything. You were in a sorority. Your coworkers probably adore you. You *scrapbook*.

Both you and your newborn little girl are gorgeous, which I know from staring at the photo on your book jacket.

You can't judge a book by its cover, or the author by the photo on the back, but I'm going to. You have social graces, boundaries and the ability to restrain yourself from saying things that come across as mean-spirited and hurtful, something you probably learned from your family of origin, not to mention years in the pageant and Greek systems. You just plain know how to act. So you might not understand blurting out something asinine.

Let me just say that at the time it was really hot in Adam's studio in a garage in Glendale and my bottled water was just out of reach and I was too self-conscious to break the mood and reach for it and one piece of my bangs kept getting in my eye and I couldn't focus. I knew my tone was wrong, that while I was trying to make myself the butt of the joke, it wasn't working. When I tried to correct it, I went to that file in my brain labeled "how to fix it when you accidentally call an entertainment reporter a c-word while trying to be self-effacing," but the file was empty. Instead, there was just a Post-it reading "Peanut butter sounds *nummy*."

Your little lime green and lavender dissertation on maternal euphoria shouldn't try my patience. So what if you write tips like "Pants with an elastic waistband are great for the first trimester"? Sure, you have a love affair with the obvious, but you are happy and productive. You had a kid and wrote a book, two things I'm struggling to do. It would be a far better thing to be the one sitting over there weeping with joy into baby Ashby's pink gingham bassinet and staring at a pile of books with your picture on the back than to be sitting over here criticizing and making fun.

There's a saying: Compare and despair. This is very true when it comes to pregnancy. There's an O'Dell around every corner, someone who just seems happier, more organized, less nauseous, more resplendent than you are. These O'Dells just seem ready to be moms.

I'm positive that there are O'Dells at every stage of motherhood.

O'Dells have short labors and wear their skinny jeans home from the hospital and O'Dells produce massive quantities of breast milk with no trouble and love every second of it. O'Dells have their moms come stay for weeks to help with the baby, because O'Dells only trust family and O'Dells just adore theirs. O'Dells teach their babies sign language and institute consistent and effective nap time routines. O'Dells make the best snacks as car pool mom, help tutor their valedictorians in high school, pack them up for college with a set of matching foot lockers in the appropriate collegiate colors and decorate their dorm rooms with both aplomb and tasteful restraint. O'Dells try not to brag about their children in medical school or modeling in Milan, but what can they do? That's just where the kids are. O'Dells get big bouquets on Mother's Day no matter where the children are in the world, because they love their mommy, but not in an overly attached, unhealthy, neurotic way. O'Dells plan their daughters' weddings without incident, and sit in the front row weeping with happiness, as they did back in the day when they had that first bout of postpartum elation. O'Dells spoil their grandchildren—though no one can believe O'Dells are actually old enough to have grandkids! O'Dells are the subject of "My Hero" essays written by their great-grandchildren. When O'Dells age, they let their hair go tastefully gray but are never, ever without manicured fingernails, painted a dusty rose. In the old folks' home, they always have more visitors than you, a steady stream who always seem to be singing. When O'Dells pass quietly and peacefully in their sleep after enjoying sixty-year marriages, their funerals are packed and the services moving. They will have a much sunnier and more expensive resting place than you will. There will always be more flowers on their graves.

It's going to be a long lifetime as a mother if I spend it feeling inferior, so I might as well get a jump on it and start now.

eight

Why I'm Finally Psyched
to Be Having a Boy

I stood in the middle of a swanky baby boutique, stuck there, as if a pink diaper pin were going right through me, fixing me to the center of the crammed little room.

It looked like a vagina had exploded in there.

There were a row of petite purses made to look like chocolate chip cookies, a set of red plastic lips containing mint lip gloss, a bubble gum pink voile skirt hanging with a dainty black cardigan, a tiara festooned with powder blue fluff. There were racks of alternating orange and yellow boas, a stack of fuchsia headbands with white dots, a giant purple flower attached to a silver hair clip and a trio of white unicorns with gold horns and eyes.

"You baby store people are totally fucking with me," I thought, my mouth hanging open so that it looked like I was having a mild stroke. Daring to glance at the boy wall, I saw one measly pair of denim overalls and a sad stack of brown Jimi Hendrix onesies.

"Can I help you?" asked the clerk.

Not unless you can turn an XY into an XX.

I was aware that it looked pretty strange, me standing there, mouth wide open, not moving, but I couldn't tell the truth, that I was pissed off about all these girlie treats I coveted for the daughter I wasn't having. So I muttered something about needing a shower gift for a little boy.

"So much cute girl stuff in here," I whispered. "Not so much boy stuff."

"Yeah, I know," chirped the saleslady, straightening a glistening display of sparkly barrettes. "Maybe some socks?"

You probably have a girl at home, saleslady, or maybe two, playing dress up as we speak or just peacefully reading a book of Emily Dickinson poems waiting for you to come home so she can tell you about her day and help you set the fucking table. You chirpy, greedy, double girl-having snatch-face.

Some socks. That's what you get when you're having a boy. If you're lucky, you scare up a tiny pair of checkered Vans, but those also serve to remind you of what he'll be wearing on his feet when he pushes toy trucks across the room, stacks piles of boring old Legos for hours and breaks everything in sight, including his own bones from time to time, trying to "fly" from the couch to the floor or playing other dubious games of his own invention. I just knew it would go from bleak brown onesies and dull blue socks with "I love Mommy" stitched to the side, to legions of army men and train sets underfoot, to a room smelling of mildew and dirty laundry and filled with hockey posters, barely used Aqua-Sport-scented deodorant sticks and one sullen, unapproachable, terse teenage boy. The last time he would say "I love Mommy" would be through his socks.

This boy would not call me much when he went off to college, or joined the merchant marine if they still have that, or whatever. He would dodge my calls, except once a week on Sundays when he would feel obliged to humor me for twenty minutes as I peppered him with annoying questions about his personal life and he gave me a series of brief, unsatisfying answers. I would never *know* him.

When he's a toddler, I wouldn't have a clue how to play with him and when he's an adult, I'd just be a nuisance until one day his new wife would suggest they move to another state and visit once a year, but only if they can stay at a hotel.

So you can see why I was paralyzed in that baby store.

That place was filled with the costumes and props from a play that would never open, starring my girl Harper and me.

Since the day I found out I was pregnant, I only saw this baby as a girl, dreamed of her daddy clumsily tying her hair in pigtails as she beamed up at me, fantasized about what I was sure would be our lifelong bond.

My girlfriend Cassandra, who is also pregnant with a boy and a few months ahead of me, is thrilled to be having a boy. "Girls? Why would you want a girl? They just get eating disorders. They're moody and bratty. Think of how we were as teenagers," she remarked, as we sat at an outdoor café drinking iced tea and eating cheese fries.

"Don't care. They're just so cute. And a girl would be your friend forever," I said.

"Wait," she paused, mid–cheese fry. "Don't you not talk to your mom?"

Oh, right. That.

And I guess I was kind of a moody teenager with an eating disorder, but still, that's the beauty of placing the responsibility for fixing your fractured childhood on your unborn baby. It doesn't have to make sense.

As facile as it seems, I think somewhere in my mind was this Barbie toy chest full of healing that would magically burst open when I did everything so much better than my mom did with me, when I taught Harper how to shave her legs and showed up to her recitals, when I bought her gauzy skirts and said things like, "I know you must be sad right now," instead of "Don't you dare manipulate me with your tears," when we wore matching Halloween costumes and had our own secret language, when she confided in me about her crushes as we sat at the kitchen table late at night, sipping hot cocoa.

Life with a daughter would be one long therapeutic spa day.

Cassandra ripped an article about "Gender Disappointment" from a magazine and gave it to me the next time I saw her. Suddenly I discovered the bargaining part of the Elisabeth Kübler-Ross stages of grief, after the shock, denial and numbness. The bargain I made with myself, with fate, was that I could get a girl *next* time. If I really needed to have a daughter, I could slip a few greenbacks in the hand of fate and give it a wink. The article covered everything from sleeping with a lime-soaked tampon to foster girl-friendly vaginal pH levels to sperm-spinning and even in vitro fertilization with preimplantation genetic diagnosis (PGD), a procedure during which only sex-identified embryos are implanted. I could have another baby, I could throw money and science at the problem, and I could have a girl. This was comforting. This is what I held on to for a week or two.

It was nice to not feel alone—most of the women quoted in the article also wanted girls—but on the other hand, these ladies made me not want to be part of their club, using their real names and often posting their suicidal boy-dreading thoughts on message boards with tips about eating kefir, berries and low-salt sesame paste to promote X sperm survival.

Clearly, I'm not one to keep my neuroses to myself, but these ladies were going on record as not being happy with their boy babies, a sentiment the grown-up boy babies could easily Google in years to come. Just as my mom thought her story about buying "It's a Boy" cards was a hilarious nugget, these girl-wanters seemed oblivious to the concept that publicizing their distaste for boys was akin to saying, "I didn't really want you. Your very existence bums me out."

So why am I telling you this?

Much like a robot would have to be programmed to convey normal human emotions (cry or frown when sad, crinkle eyes with big smile when happy), I have to be told how to maintain normal human boundaries, how to know the difference between revealing an embarrassing weakness that might make for a compelling story and telling a hurtful secret that would cause irreparable harm. My impulse has always been to tell, tell, tell my ass off and hope that someone will relate, and maybe empathize, and maybe like me a little more for my brokenness and candor.

In this case, my therapist recommended that I not talk about it on the radio or write about it in my blog. She straightened me out the way a parent explains to a five-year-old that it isn't nice to announce to the fat lady on the bus that she's fat.

"Yeah, you should only talk about this in here," she warned. "Your son might find out, and that's bad."

"Really? Oh, right. Right. Okay. That would be bad. Thank you," I said, nodding and vowing to stick to the phrase she gave me, even in conversations with friends, the one that isn't a lie but doesn't tell the whole truth: "A girl would be nice eventually, but I'm really excited about *this* boy."

The more I say it, the truer it becomes. And I wouldn't be writing about this now if the longing for a girl hadn't lifted, or maybe just passed through me like a nasty flu.

The girl craving that peaked that day in the boutique and threatened to undo me is gone, and I'm not really sure how it dissolved so completely other than the phrase "my boy."

I just like the sound of it, the vision of me walking through my front door after work and asking, "Where's my boy?" This vision extends to me showing up at day care to pick him up and asking, "How did my boy do today?" It branches into imagining the family gearing up for a road trip, me asking my husband, "Have you packed up the boy?" The boy. My boy. Our boy. All three are starting to sound right to me.

What really sings to me is this idea, possibly revolting in its cheesiness: I will be referring to my son and his father as "my boys." I'll phone home from the freeway to ask if "my boys" need me to pick anything up for dinner. "I need a hug from my boys," I'll announce on a Sunday morning, over coffee and the paper.

Maybe I have Stockholm syndrome. I have fallen in love with my little captor because I have no choice: This fetus has a penis. Either way, I am so good with this boy thing right now.

Boys grow up to carry their mother's luggage (not the emotional baggage I was hoping Harper would tote, but actual Samsonite). They give gangly boy hugs to their mothers. They fall asleep with toy airplanes in their hands because they don't want to put them down, want to dream about flying. They shyly ask their moms advice about girls. Or maybe my boy will like other boys, and original-cast albums of Broadway shows, and that will be fine, too, because maybe my girl would pull a Chastity Bono on me anyway, and not strictly adhere to the gender clichés, hating ribbons and bows and begging to watch the guy at the hardware store make a key.

This idea tickles me more than that rack of boas would: I may have accidentally started being a decent parent already, because I've already stopped counting on this boy to make it all better. I don't know which way he's going, but I'm squatted down with a low center of gravity, ready to go any direction, ready to follow his lead. I'm ready to love the hell out of this boy, not for what he can do for me but for how fun it might be to get to know him.

The more I think about that magazine article, the battier and crueler those women seem, and I'm flooded with relief. The feeling didn't pass because I'm superior, or because I did anything magical to get rid of it, or because I'm destined for maternal greatness. It just passed.

I still don't know much about boys.

I just know that this one, my boy, is crowding my diaphragm, lungs and stomach, while simultaneously making room in my heart. I hate that I even wrote that sentence, but the pregnancy hormones are robbing me of my ability to be cynical sometimes. I have to do crazy shit like talk about my fucking heart, but at least cursing makes me feel less vulnerable and stupid about it. Fucking heart.

People I Want to Punch: Great Sleeper People

Great sleepers can sleep anywhere, and they can't shut up about it.

Here's what you sound like, sleepyheads: *"I sleep in the car! I sleep standing up! I sleep on a pile of coats at a party! I sleep while operating a jackhammer! I fall asleep on the toilet sometimes! I sleep in the break room at the office! Does coffee keep me up? Heck no. I enjoy a strong espresso after dinner every night and I nod right off. Sometimes, I actually hit my head right on the tiny mug. I just love sleeping. I could sleep eleven hours a night. If I don't get at least eight hours, I'm a mess. If you're tired, why don't you just take a nap?"*

Sleepers can't grasp insomnia. As well rested as they are, you'd think they would have ready access to empathy. Instead, advising us to take naps is like telling a depressive to just "cheer up." They're simply not tuned in to those of us with psyches that refuse to let us relax.

If your brain has an on-off switch, mine has a choir. The altos sing a to-do list, the tenors are belting out words to an e-mail I shouldn't have written, the sopranos are reminding me to think about cutting out dairy, the bass provides a steady thrum of self-doubt, la la la, self-doubt, la la la, while the soloist sings, "Are we the only mammals who know that we die?" In the mind of the easy sleeper: old-school slow jams or a medley of Celtic harp music. While we have a crescendo choir of assholes we can't turn down, you might even have total silence, or an internal Sharper Image white-noise machine set on ocean waves. Explaining chronic insomnia to great sleepers is like explaining Thomas Pynchon to a toddler. He isn't going to grasp *Gravity's Rainbow*. That's why great sleepers, instead of learning an important lesson called Nodding Sympathetically While Saying, "I know this must be hard," suggest herb tea, sleep masks and naps. *Naps*.

You don't just sleep—you make a spectacle of your repose by snoring, drooling, looking extra cozy and sleeping in the most awkward positions imaginable. You doze without a blanket in a chilly room, your bare feet mocking my need for ideal sleep conditions. You sleep with your head mashed against a scratchy couch, pressing a tweed pattern into your cheeks. You snooze through fire alarms and earthquakes. You siesta peacefully after getting fired or dumped, and you have no trouble falling immediately into a deep slumber the night before taking a big exam, starting a new job, or getting a kidney transplant.

As far back as I can remember, sleeping was something I knew normal people did with ease and regularity.

Little girls with pink rooms and white wicker beds whose mommies tucked them into bed with warm milk and animal crackers, those little bitches put their pigtails on the gingham pillowcase and it was *nighty-night*. I had been to enough slumber parties and sleepovers to know that little worried freaks like me with freaky thoughts were probably the only ones awake in the middle of the night.

Even as a seven-year-old, I would get in bed and stare at the ceiling for hours, my mind racing. I remember worrying about whether I had cavities, concerned that at my dentist appointment in three months the hygienist would narc me out for eating sugar, which my hippie parents didn't allow me to have. They would just know I had been eating SweeTarts and fun-size Charleston Chews from the look of my tooth enamel, and I would have some explaining to do about all of my lying. This is the kind of issue that seemed so pressing that I had to imagine the many ways it might play out, just as I had to imagine the multitude of angles from which the bogeyman could strike, causing me to gnash my surely rotting teeth.

While other children were enjoying sleep, one of the most basic of human needs, I would reenact conversations with the girls at ballet school that hadn't gone well, or consider the odds that my grandpa would have a heart attack and drop dead before I could apologize for spilling nail polish remover on his tax returns.

As you can imagine, once caffeinated beverages and puberty entered the picture, it only got worse.

When I think about college, I think about watching Charlie Rose interview various obscure notables on my tiny black-and-white television propped up on a milk crate. When "The Star-Spangled Banner" came on, I would switch to news radio. Traffic, weather, news, traffic, weather, news, trying not to check the clock, checking the clock, endless calculations about how much sleep I would get if I just fell asleep *now*. Or now. Or now. Or within fifteen minutes from now. Or this hour.

Under ideal conditions, when the temperature is moderate, the bedding clean and fluffy, the room neat and the life situation calm, I still have to read or watch television before falling asleep. Pregnancy, with its attendant physical discomforts and emotionally charged future projections, is me teaching a master class on insomnia to Mr. Sandman.

Good sleeper people, you mean well, but you all seem to think if you can't get a good night's sleep, you should just nap. You never shut up about the merits of goddamn napping, as though somehow it's easier to sleep in the middle of the day.

Here's you: *"You should just nap. I love naps. Just a twenty-minute snooze makes me feel so refreshed. I just put on my sleep mask and out I go."*

Just the thought of you in REM as I struggle to find a position that doesn't squish my swollen boobs or

jostle my constantly full bladder, just the idea of you log-
ging a full night of rest makes me jealous and resentful.
Good sleeper people, especially those of you who are
also pregnant and should really be spending the wee
hours flipping through pregnancy books to see what
symptoms you can expect every week until your due
date, you are as irritating as the red numbers on a digital clock flashing all night long.

On top of the usual strain of being awake when the
world has stopped, I now have to worry that I am
stressing out my tiny fetus with my insomnia and the
worries that cause it. I have a new pastime as I readjust
my pillow for the forty-seventh time: Instead of counting
sheep, I count the ways I want to punch you good
sleepers, and put you to sleep for a good long time.

First Trimester Box Score

Here is my current pregnancy stat sheet.
Just remember, not everything is in the numbers. This pregnancy has big upside potential. Lots of hustle. Maybe I'll get scouted to deliver in the minors.

STRASSER'S ROOKIE SEASON ON THE BABY BREWERS

2   hemorrhoids

2   bladder infections

39   years of age

3.6   emotional breakdowns

5   missed work meetings and therapy appointments due to pregnancy confusion, or "baby brain"

3 instances of locking myself out of the house in my pajamas

2 bra cup size increases

67 times I've Googled the word "miscarriage" in combination with various behavior or symptoms

4 sonograms

1 first-trimester screening

1 CVS test

2 genetic disorders found in my DNA

3 full bottles of Cherry Mylanta consumed

1 bottle Zantac prescribed (useless)

1 bottle Zofran prescribed (useless)

5 baby names in the running, none really grabbing me

1 shaming yoga teacher who announced, "This should be your last regular class. Prenatal yoga is on Tuesdays." Namaste to you, too, m-fer.

1 extreme full-body acne outbreak

12 containers Fage yogurt consumed between hours of twelve and three a.m.

9 cups frozen grapes consumed between hours of twelve and three a.m.

16 hours of *This American Life* downloaded for listening pleasure in the bathtub during the dark, scary nighttime hours

4   tubs powdered organic bubble bath used

27 spins of the Talking Heads song "Stay Up Late."
    Little pee-pee, little toes.

17 proclamations about my future boy, including, "He
    is going to love reading. And hate binge drinking."

2   moments I stopped cold walking on the sidewalk.
    Paused. Had to stand still to really consider: What
    have I gotten myself into?

nine

How Freaky and Paranoid Is Your Google History?

This is almost like "found poetry," if you found a really depressing and sparsely written poem. Here is a verbatim history of my baby-related Google searches for my third month of pregnancy. How do you describe obsessive, all-consuming anxiety? Like they say in Comp 101: Show, don't tell.

Miscarriage signs

Baby book Spock[1]

Toddler Guitar

Beer and pregnancy

Guinness beer good for you BBC

Guinness beer iron[2]

---

[1]Never bought it, maybe not enough scaremongering for me. "Trust yourself, you know more than you think you do"? Um, you don't know me, dude.

[2]Apparently, this stout does seem to contain some iron and was therefore once thought of as a health tonic excellent for pregnant or nursing women. Then again, you could get more iron from an egg, and not risk fetal alcohol syndrome, but who quibbles with tradition?

Beer and pregnancy

O'Doul's pregnancy safe?

Imminent miscarriage

Emergen-C pregnancy safe

Hot baths pregnancy neural tube defects

Is it safe to take a hot bath while pregnant?

Hot baths: safe during pregnancy?

Pregnancy—Birth: Cause of miscarriage

Does anyone still take hot baths?

Pregnancy and baby: Are hot baths safe?

The myths and facts about pregnancy

Stretch mark cream reviews

Imminent miscarriage

Stretch mark product reviews[3]

Reviews of top five stretch mark remover creams

The Doctor's Book of Home Remedies: stretch marks

Octo-Mom: "I was a stripper"

CVS: chorionic villus sampling

Discharge normal after CVS

CVS cramps villus

CVS prenatal diagnosis

Fitness for Two: March of Dimes

According to my Google research on this topic, Guinness has no more iron than any other beer. My craving remains unexplained.

[3] A note on stretch mark obsession: People tell me not to worry because stretch marks are genetic. Too bad I'm worried because my mom has terrible stretch marks.

Braxton Hicks CVS after

Braxton Hicks contractions

First trimester screening

CVS not risky?

Imminent miscarriage[4]

Miscarriage

What brings on miscarriage?

Preventing miscarriage

Life after miscarriage

Nonviable pregnancy but no miscarriage yet

Abnormal first trimester screening results

CVS testing and miscarriage

First trimester screening negative results

CVS miscarriage

CVS test

CVS test reliability

CVS, not the pharmacy

Nonalcoholic beer during pregnancy

O'Doul's alcohol content[5]

Ampicillin—nausea bladder

Ampicillin nausea

---

[4]Proof that we don't live in an Orwellian society reminiscent of *Nineteen Eighty-Four*: If there really was some kind of Internet oversight happening, you know, looking for insurgents who Google things like "where to buy fertilizer," Big Brother would have come after me for the number of times I Google "miscarriage."

[5]Finally broke down and drank half a nonalcoholic beer. None of the great taste, all of the guilt. Rest of six-pack still in fridge.

CVS Cedars-Sinai

Fucking CVS

Imminent miscarriage

Prenatal 3D ultrasound safety issues

Are new ultrasound technologies causing autism?

Sonogram autism[6]

Baby sucking thumb on ultrasound

Pregnancy and baby: ultrasound

It's a boy for Carson Daly and girlfriend[7]

Ellen Pompeo pregnant

Pompeo baby weight

Lady from Grey's Anatomy skinny

Ashlee Simpson baby weight

How old is Ashlee Simpson?

Young women baby weight

Urinary tract infections

Positive urine nitrate test

Enterococcus bladder infection catheter

Bladder infection: information from Answers.com

---

[6]Thank you, Jenny McCarthy. No, I'm not being sarcastic. I think it's great that you raised awareness. However, I wish it wasn't raised quite so high right now. I'm starting to envy our parents, who thought autism was a nineteenth-century painting style. This is all we pregnant girls are hearing about and there isn't much we can do about it until we have to figure out the vaccine thing, so it really is just one of those things you Google for a month and then just say fuck it. You are no wiser for all your Googling, but have wasted some of your precious time on this earth.

[7]Suddenly other people having babies becomes interesting even if they are not inherently interesting.

Mantras for letting go[8]

Celebrities with first name: Mick

Celebrities with first name: Shane

Imminent miscarriage

The Mommy Files: 7 superfoods you should be eating

Prenatal vitamins make me sick

Fetal movement: feeling your baby kick

Fitness/nutrition: your first trimester: iVillage

Best camcorder

Imminent miscarriage

What your baby looks like—10 weeks—babycenter

Do you want to know your baby's gender?

Caffeine during pregnancy

Sleep aids during pregnancy[9]

Exposure to oral contraceptives and risk for Down syndrome

Folate and human development

Down syndrome likelihood 38

Causes of Down syndrome

Risk factors for Down syndrome

Loving a child with Down syndrome

Best physician Los Angeles[10]

9 weeks pregnant?

---

[8]You can see from my single Googling of this that I quickly let go of trying to let go.

[9]Dead end. Count sheep.

[10]Looking up doctors on review sites like Yelp is useful mainly if you enjoy nasty, bitter people venting about rude receptionists.

Showing pregnancy

First pregnancy and showing early

Gestational diabetes

Diabetes and birth weight

Organic frosting

Healthy sweeteners cupcakes Los Angeles

Me hungry

What is the meaning of life?

Oldest mother on record British

When can babies hear music

Reflux, food, causes

Constipation pregnancy iron

Most expensive stretch mark cream

Pregnancy exercise linked to high IQ

Latest week pregnancy miscarriage risk

Pregnancy gallery: 10 weeks[11]

Treadmill pregnancy safe

Short torso and pregnancy

Lasers to treat stretch marks

Ideal temperature bath pregnancy

Hot bath and pregnancy

Wikianswers: hot bath and gin end pregnancy

---

[11]Pregnancy galleries are generally badly lit belly shots that look like amateur porn, but serve to help you compare your size to other nameless pregnant ladies on the Web.

Expecting? Pregnancy myths exposed

Gender prediction

The truth about gender prediction

Imminent miscarriage

People.com: Strasser expecting first baby[12]

---

[12] Okay, so I Googled myself!

ten

Logan's Running

I order a smoothie and the man doesn't offer me a free boost.

"Can I get a Vitabek?" I ask.

"Umm. Those aren't good for pregnant girls."

And this is the first time someone, totally unprovoked, alludes to the baby. Just from looking at me.

Which makes today one of those days I know for sure that I'm pregnant.

This isn't just something I want to be true. This isn't just some ruse my doctor and husband are in on, cooking up fake sonograms just to make me happy and using some other baby's prerecorded heartbeat sound to convince me.

The confused background processing that passes for thinking in the pregnant mind can present this as a real possibility: Every symptom, every item of clothing that no longer fits, every middle-of-the-night leg cramp, every esophagus-scorching bout of heartburn, these are all just figments, coincidences. Maybe a delusion, an elaborate sham, or a long trance.

There can't really be a *baby*.

That would be too weird, if you just wanted to have a baby, had unprotected sex, and two months later peed on a stick and got a plus sign. That could not have happened. Not to me.

Yet this smoothie guy is a total stranger. He could not be in on the hoax. He took one look at me and decided it would be a bad idea to offer me a boost. Because I'm *pregnant*. I tell him I think the vitamin boost will probably be okay, and he says he didn't want to say anything to me because last time he declined to give someone a boost, the lady turned out not to be pregnant and he felt terrible about insulting her. I check out the reflection of my belly's profile in the glass door of the smoothie shop and announce, "Well, I really am pregnant, so don't feel bad."

And the most banal of errands, just running out to get a raspberry banana smoothie, turns out to be pretty juicy. (Carrie Bradshaw just vomited when she read that last line. Give me a break. They can't all be gems.)

Emboldened by the fact that even the smoothie guy knows I'm pregnant, I clutch my giant vitamin-enhanced beverage and wander, finding myself at a park on Beverly Boulevard near Larchmont Village. I've never been here before, though I've driven by a thousand times, barely registering the balloons on the picnic tables, swing sets, jungle gyms. Maybe I just want to get close to where the mom people and children go. There are strollers, sippy cups, nannies and a playground lousy with toddlers.

Spreading out my sweater on the grass, I survey the scene for a second, and wonder if this is home, or the future, or an oasis of simple pleasures I don't yet understand, or some kind of grape juice–stained, soul-crushing daily drudgery that I will never, ever embrace or even hack. I look for signs, read the mom faces. I give up, deciding I have five more months to figure it out. I return a few calls. I download a meditation app on my iPhone and zone out, which is easier now than ever. Pregnancy hormones are supposed to be making me overwrought and insane, but I started out that way, so perhaps they are having the opposite effect. Being in the second trimester feels like being stoned; I'm forgetful, unmotivated, want to eat strange food combinations and just feel high. First-trimester angst has largely given way to a mind-set not unlike an early Eagles song, peaceful and easy, allowing me to smash my previous meditation record of three and a half minutes.

When I come to, a woman is screaming at an old man in a straw hat and faded plaid shirt. "Don't talk to these kids. Get out of here. You are disgusting and you should be ashamed of yourself."

She is pointing at his face and there is a chorus of silent moms behind her, arms crossed, chinos in a bunch, angry, but no one calls 911. I don't know what the story is with these moms and this old man. I want to help, but I feel detached, like I'm observing the whole thing behind glass in a mom exhibit somewhere.

The old man swivels on the bench, which is oriented toward the playground. He turns sideways, head on his shoulder, and stares right at me. *I am way too old for you, pal.* Maybe he's trying to get a gander at my tiny, naked fetus. Creepy. Now I have to worry about registered sex offenders, or I guess it's really the unregistered sex offenders that should concern me. Maybe this guy is just a geezer who enjoys the bench on a sunny afternoon, I don't know. I don't know whose side I'm on, but visiting the park is like taking a college tour when you can't picture leaving home but know your departure is looming. Some of the park moms seem bored and some seem put-upon and others seem quietly content. Some have nannies with them and some swing their children with one hand and tie their hair back with the other. All of them seem much older and more mature than I am (though let's face it, most are probably younger), but even the smoothie guy knows that I'm about to be one of them. I may be rubbernecking now, but it won't be long before I'm living life in the mom lane, which will surely make me lose my mind. Or not. For now, I can just Take It Easy.

There were moms and babies all around before; I just never noticed them. Now, I carefully observe them everywhere I go, stare at a woman struggling to corral her little boy at the grocery store while attaching her infant's car seat to the top of her cart. The diaper and baby food aisle has always been there, but I've never walked down it until now. The bulletin board at the bagel shop has always been covered with ads for Mommy and Me classes and babysitters, but now I take note. It's not that baby stores are sprouting up at strip malls across the greater Los Angeles area; it's just that I can finally see what's always been there.

Being pregnant for the first time is like learning a new word; suddenly you hear it all the time, now that you finally know what it means.

Will I go to this very park with my boy? Stroll him to the smoothie shop so I can show him off to the smoothie man and reassure him the vitamin boost was okay? Will I know how to play with him, seeing as I've never pushed a child on a swing in my life, or handled a sippy cup, diaper or onesie? Will I be accepted into this clan of moms? Do babies need sunscreen or just a hat? What if caring for a child is so gratifying that I never want to work again? Or, what if, like my mother, I will take any job I can get to afford paying a nanny to do all of this for me? If there is a continuum of mommy excellence, with Medea on one end and June Cleaver on the other, where will I land? Hopefully, nowhere near Nancy O'Dell, who owes me a punch in the face, though I assume she is pretty close to June Cleaver in overall saintliness.

It's cooling off, but I stay even after the old guy bails. A mom in a striped oxford and Keds ties the ends of a knit hat under the chin of her wriggly child and produces a box of raisins from somewhere in her giant backpack. Some kid trips and cries. Every kid seems to be named Logan. "Logan, say you're sorry. Logan, you want your juice box? Logan, I said stop that. Logan, time to go. Logan, I said time to go. Logan, it's okay, play nice. Logan, do you remember your friend Logan? You met him last week. *Logan!!!! Not on the slide!* Logan, tell your brother Logan to put on his sweater because we have to go. Logan, you need a nap. Logan, this is what happens when you eat candy. Logan, this is what happens when you don't go pee before we leave the house. Logan, use your words. Logan, don't be shy. Logan, don't run. Logan, say good-bye to Logan, Logan and Logan."

A quick search on the iPhone reveals that the name Logan is of Scottish and Gaelic origin and means "hollow." A baby name Web site explains that the name gained momentum in recent years, a fact the site attributes to the character Brooke Logan on *The Bold and the Beautiful*. Really? A word meaning "hollow" becomes ubiquitous at a Los Angeles park because of a soap opera character who has a brother named Storm and a romantic history with a guy named Ridge (more Googling).

It's almost dark now, and the moms have scattered and I realize that there is a lot of information I just don't have yet and a lot of it you can't get on your iPhone. I toss my spent smoothie in the trash. I stare at the abandoned playground, pull the sleeves of my sweater over my hands. I'm stuck here motionless for a second, with no one to tell me if I'll ever want to come back, or if I'll ever belong, or if my mom days at the park will be filled with wonder or Valium. There is no way to know if the future will be like a never-ending, poorly reviewed science fiction movie or if I will enjoy watching the Logans run.

eleven

The Ten Worst Moms in History

At five months pregnant, I think a lot about Ruth Bader Ginsburg. It's not just that she's the second woman ever to be appointed to the Supreme Court of the United States, but also because with her prim lace collars, understated pearl earrings and overall vibe of measured thoughtfulness and calm, she seems like a great mom. I wish she were my mom sometimes. I don't know the woman, but I even kind of wish she could be my child's mom. Who wouldn't want to climb up on that robed lap and hear about how Mom volunteered for the ACLU or learned a new language to coauthor a book on judicial procedure in Sweden?

It's not just Ruth. There are many women, famous and not, who seem much better suited for the job of motherhood.

There are times I feel sorry for my unborn child, because he will have me for a mother, and not someone more calm and together.

Kids need to be reassured that everything is okay, whereas my general opinion is that the sky is falling and everyone hates me. I don't just sweat the small stuff, I flop sweat it.

I regularly miss ten freeway off-ramps just crafting a paragraph in my head or memorizing lines, after which I come to and panic because I'm horribly lost. I regularly leave the curling iron on until it singes the dresser and any nearby hand towels. So far, I've exhibited no patience for learning about birthing, birthing centers or baby development. When my doctor was running half an hour behind, I didn't think, "Oh, well, I'll just use this time to quietly reflect on this beautiful transition," but instead, I approached the receptionist seventeen times to whisper, "ETA?" After that, I sat there angrily flipping the pages of *American Cheerleader* magazine and rolling my eyes. Kids don't like eye rollers. They need someone who can go with the flow.

I'm not a leaf in the stream, but a coagulated hunk of hair and soap clogging your drain.

When I think about the fact that my baby is stuck with someone as imperfect as me for his primary female caregiver, I get so down there is nothing to do but focus on women who I think would be or have been way, way worse. It's astonishing—and a bit sad, frankly—how much compiling an inventory of inferior moms puts me at ease. All I can say is that coming up with this kind of list makes me feel better about my own mom potential. So, with all due respect, thank you, worst moms in history, for lowering the bar.

JOANNA KRAMER—This mother, played by Meryl Streep in the 1979 film *Kramer vs. Kramer*, represented all that was wrong with '70s moms. Joanna—icy, selfish and beleaguered—bails on her family, only to return a year and a half later to take back her son and screw up the life he's finally put together with his pops, played by Dustin Hoffman. She wins little Billy back after a character-assassinating custody battle, but in the end, decides, whoops, sorry, he's better off with his dad. It was all so harrowing that Justin Henry, who played Billy, got an Oscar nomination, becoming the youngest actor to earn that distinction.

With her chunky leather boots, neck scarves and patrician cheekbones, Joanna brought glamour to maternal abandonment.

"All my life I've felt like somebody's wife or somebody's mother or somebody's daughter. Even all the time we were together, I never knew who I was. And that's why I had to go away. And in California, I think I found myself," says Joanna, explaining why she left her kid. Can you feel her pain? Boo hoo!

Of course, Joanna Kramer is emblematic of that whole generation of moms, because they always put a premium on "finding themselves." This was such an important pursuit in the '70s that lots of moms, like JK, were able to find themselves only by losing their kids. Thus, the second wave of feminism crashed hard on some kids, and you know you're one if you can't watch the scene in which Dustin Hoffman pleads for his kid in court without shedding a tear.

When little Billy asks, "When's Mommy coming back?" it breaks our spirits first broken by our broken homes.

The movie struck such a chord that it cleaned up at the Academy Awards, winning Best Picture and garnering Best Actress and Best Actor awards for Streep and Hoffman.

Now fictional Joanna Kramer, who represents so many cold, bored, motherhood-isn't-for-me moms, wins this important honor, one of the worst mothers in history.

MRS. WOLF SPIDER—A bad mother might not make her children lunch, but a worse mother might actually *make her children lunch*. What I mean is, a mama wolf spider is generally harmless, unless you happen to be her baby wolf spider. Once born, the babies congregate on their mother's stomach, ready to be fed. In some cases, however, they wind up being the mother's next meal instead. It's one thing if your mother resented you, or read your diary, or spent all of her time with your alcoholic stepfather, or just never "got" you, but it's another thing if she decided you were more delicious than adorable.

Zoologists have a tough time explaining filial cannibalism, the act of eating one's offspring. One theory is that it roots out the weakest of the young, those that are taking too long to mature and would require more parental care. Theoretically, if the wolf spider mom eats the worst of her little wolf spiders, she will have more energy for superior ones.

Talk about pressure.

MARILU HENNER—I feel a bit harsh putting this beloved actress on the list of worst moms. I mean, all she did was write a parenting book, *I Refuse to Raise a Brat*, and plaster her two sons, Nicholas and Joseph, on the cover. Personally, I would hate to have my mother's literary career and overall cred depend on my ability to keep my shit together at the grocery store, at recess, at day care and everywhere prying eyes were looking for signs that I was, in fact, a brat.

As if that wasn't enough, Marilu followed up her brat book by penning *Healthy Kids*, which warns against the dangers of "dead food" and instructs parents to avoid sugar, chemicals, dairy and anything else a kid might want to eat.

So to review, her kids could not be bratty or chubby, nor could they ever eat a marshmallow in public. Then again, as Marilu writes, "Children must learn that they can't always get their way."

That is definitely what they'll learn in elementary school trying to trade their mung beans and rice for a box of Red Vines. "Their way" will be kale salad with gluten-free dressing eaten with chopsticks at the lonely corner of the playground. All because Mommy already spent the first third of the advance for the second book and needed to immediately expand her field of expertise to child nutrition. Nothing tastes worse than being the house on the block that gives out toothbrushes and lectures on Halloween.

Your food may be "alive," but with this mom, you'll wish you weren't.

Sorry, Elaine Nardo. Loved you on *Celebrity Apprentice*, and you seem like a nice lady, but you went from exploiting your kids, which I endorse, to setting them up to fail as shining examples of your child-rearing philosophies. Maybe they'll turn out to be amazingly well-adjusted and wonderful men, but that doesn't mean you didn't ruin their childhoods with a combo platter of rigidity and carob.

MEDEA—This one is a gimme. Or more of a takey, as in, takey your own kids' lives. You gotta go mythological for a mother this venal. In Euripides' famous play based on the Greek myth, Jason leaves his wife, Medea, for a princess. Medea, in turn, butchers their two sons with a knife. Granted, it sucks to be left for a princess, but killing your kids for revenge means you will always make this list. And when someone like Susan Smith or Andrea Yates kills her kids, your name is going to come up until the end of time.

Here is your challenge, ladies: Find a way of getting revenge without killing the kids.

For example, Lisa "Left Eye" Lopes famously burned football player Andre Rison's house to the ground. Simple, effective—point made, plenty of headlines, no kids harmed. There are so many ways to open up a can of crazy and make a man regret cheating on you without filicide. By the way, though it's been done all over the world, I don't recommend cutting off his penis, strictly on the grounds that it lacks poetry. Or, I should say, the poetry is a bit on the nose and you don't want your revenge gesture to be as trite as it is grisly.

Medea really got Jason where it hurt, but among other flaws with her historic act, it's hard to go back and do that one again. You play that hand once, and then what do you do for an encore? Kill his cousins?

Sure, ancient Greece was a rough psychological neighborhood, but Medea managed to stand out even in that crowd.

I bet if she had held off for a few months, she probably would have realized Jason wasn't even all that. She would have dropped a few pounds from the heartache and popped over to the oracle to scope out some single guys wearing her "skinny" tunic and a new pair of sandals. Maybe she could have found an ancient friend with benefits or a support group of other single Argonaut divorcées.

What do I know, but it seems being a mom means protecting your kids, not making them the ultimate "burn on you."

DEMI MOORE—It's not her fault, but no matter how old she gets, Demi Moore is probably going to be hotter than her three beautiful daughters. I file Demi with Naomi Judd, Cybill Shepherd and Christie Brinkley under "painfully pretty moms," who can't help but cast a big beautiful shadow over their daughters. And as we all know from Bette Midler, shadows are cold, they are cold dank places to catch eating disorders and while away hours studying one's pores in a hand mirror.

It pains me to include Demi on this list, because there is so much to love about one of America's premier MILFs. Aside from her hardscrabble upbringing and alcoholic parents, she struck just the right tone with her baby exploiting when she famously posed nude and seven months pregnant with daughter Scout LaRue, bringing attention not only to herself and her career (good job), but also celebrating pregnant women everywhere as sex symbols.

Yet therein lies the problem. Demi looked hot in her third trimester, she looked hot with a shaved head in *G.I. Jane*, she looked hot pre–boob job in *About Last Night*, she looked hot in what should have been an unflattering navy uniform in *A Few Good Men*. She looked almost impossibly hot at forty in *Charlie's Angels: Full Throttle*, and from what I can tell from paparazzi photos, when she and Ashton Kutcher frolic on various beaches, she still looks just as hot in her bikini. One day, she may stop being hot, but I can't imagine that day. I just can't. Even her voice is hot.

We can't blame her for possessing enduring beauty, but it might be nice if she would dowdy it up a little bit or maybe ease up on the plastic surgery and yoga, rock a St. John's knit once in a while, allow a wrinkle to take hold. Instead, she refuses to age. She recently credited her youthful appearance to "laughter," so I have to assume her surgeon is fucking hilarious. Moreover, while other moms are referring to iPods as "machines" and generally losing touch with technology, Demi is flirting with her husband via Twitter, so the entire Twitterverse can enjoy when Ashton sends millions of followers a photo of his wife's perfect ass. That's all fine, except his wife is her kids' *mom*, and now her exquisiteness is inescapable across multiple media platforms.

Again, I'm sorry. I feel for anyone with a broken childhood and she gets extra points for wearing giant nerdy glasses as a kid and overall coming across like a loving and fiercely protective mother. Still, would I want photos of my mom's flawless ass seen by the entire world as they inevitably compare me to her? Every single time I hear that Righteous Brothers' song from *Ghost*, do I want to remember that Mom will always be a hair (a perfectly straightened and coiffed hair) prettier? The only thing more Unchained than the Melody would be my identity crisis.

TERRIE PETRIE—You may remember her from Dr. Baden's HBO documentary series *Autopsy*. This befuddled Canadian mom wrote to Dr. Baden for help. First, her eight-day-old daughter died of SIDS, and later her three-month-old twins also died of SIDS. Only, they didn't, according to Dr. Baden. After a long investigation, the forensic pathologist concluded that Terrie, who was sleeping with her twins after going out for a few cocktails, managed to roll over both times and smother them. Terrie was disappointed when she got the "cause of death" news, because she was kind of crossing her fingers for "genetic abnormality."

Let it be said, these are examples not of world-class bad people but of horrifyingly bad mommying. Hence, Terrie makes the grade by soaring to new levels of neglect. I mean, fool me once, shame on you, fool me twice—you know what I'm saying? This lady accidentally smothered three kids. Accidents happen and I can't imagine the guilt and despair, but you would think after the first unfortunate smothering that this gal might buy one of those cosleeper things, or perhaps a freakin' crib.

KATE GOSSELIN—Forget the usual stuff people hate about Kate; none of that lands her on this list. For me, it's the eight little plates of hummus and sliced apples, the matching outfits, the annoying attention to maternal detail. Kate just overmoms it. While most of the worst moms in history got there by under-momming it, Kate represents all of the women who make the rest of the moms feel inadequate. Overmoms do things like grimly interview a dozen pediatricians before choosing the one that she deems best, no matter how far from her home; they blend their own organic baby food after weekly visits to the farmer's market; they carry pacifier wipes in neatly packed and coordinated diaper bags, and generally tackle motherhood with all of the unfettered joy of a maximum-security prison warden.

Overmoms act like they are doing all of this for their children, when it's usually just one long, vain, self-serving performance. Kate happens to be known for her work on television, but she represents an army of overmoms whose audience may be the in-laws or the neighbors, or all the other parents at school who have to receive her personally hand-knit birthday invitations.

Plus, her overmommying extended to overwifing, infantilizing her ex-husband until you almost pictured him in an Ed Hardy onesie sucking a pacifier in a car seat waiting for her to change his poopy diaper and shame him for not knowing how to use the potty. If part of mothering is modeling a halfway decent marital relationship, Kate also gets points for treating her ex like a valet.

She had to have known what she was doing when she chose an easily overshadowed *shmo* like Jon. She put this third-rate IT nerd through her parenting boot camp, emasculated him with her epic bossiness, and will now keep the mommying spotlight on herself until those eight kids run away screaming. To their own reality shows, no doubt.

DR. RUTH—America desperately needed Dr. Ruth. And Dr. Ruth is a hero. I just don't know if I want my mom talking about G-spots, multiple orgasms, masturbation, premature ejaculation, proper condom usage, menstruation, or the dangers of rough anal sex. In a word: eeeewwww. I love that Dr. Ruth exists, but to be the child of the woman whose name is synonymous with frank sex talk must be kind of rough—not as rough as the anal sex she says can be risky, but rough.

As someone whose mother often disturbed me with her sexual openness, I know how uncomfortable it can be to hear your mom say anything sexual. But Ruth Westheimer doesn't just discuss sex on radio and television; she's written lots of sex books, including an actual encyclopedia of sexuality, a guidebook on sex for women over fifty, a treatise on "erotic pleasures" and even *Dr. Ruth's Guide to Talking About Herpes.*

"What's your mom do?"

"Um. She's . . . um. Do you know how the weather is supposed to be today? I heard it might rain."

It might rain a shower of Mom's herpes book on you, if the other kids find out and have a library card. If Dr. Ruth is your mom, you can be very proud, but not too proud to shorten your last name to West and head that direction away from anyone who can trace your lineage back to your real mom.

OCTOMOM—Creepy? Check. Attention-seeking? Check. Dishonest, delusional and superbly oblivious about her children's well-being? Check, check and check. Octomom gets bonus bad mom points for attracting the likes of fuchsia-lipped Gloria Allred, who scares children as much as she scares opposing counsel.

Nadya Suleman, an unemployed single mother of six who added to her brood by having octuplets using in vitro fertilization, is such an easy target that I was tempted to skip her, but that would make this whole list suspect.

Not only does the Octomom seem to be filling some deep psychological hole by continuing to have babies she can't afford, she also seems like a compulsive liar and media hound. And there's the question one always asks the mother of multiples: With that many kids, how can you possibly exploit each one of them equally?

Getting lost in the shuffle would actually be a best-case scenario for an octo-kid, because a day out with Mom at Disneyland means fighting for camera time while you get ignored in favor of any digital recording device.

JOAN CRAWFORD—"No wire hangers" is as famous an awful

mom line as there is. Whether *Mommie Dearest* is totally factual or just the narrow way Joan's daughter, Christina, recalls her childhood doesn't matter now, because Joan is the subject of a kitsch classic and is inextricably linked to the campiest maternal fit captured on film. The eyebrows, the image obsession, the succession of boyfriends Christina had to call "uncle" and the daughter-annihilating, scenery-chewing meltdowns forever cement Joan in the collective consciousness as one of history's worst mothers.

Ultimately, one of the worst things you can be called in the world is a terrible mother. There's a special ring in public relations hell for bad moms. I've been through my own mother situation, and the last thing I want is to be anywhere near this list.

These women took the hits, and sometimes gave them, so the rest of us could have some perspective. Maybe I'll take a wrong tone in explaining how the tooth fairy doesn't exist, maybe I'll send you to school with mismatched socks, maybe I won't be helpful with civics homework, but listen, future child: I won't drown you, smother you, abandon you, thwack you with wire hangers, eat you, mortify you with talk of herpetic lesions or marry Jon Gosselin. If I can avoid those things, I'll basically be doing all right. While it's inevitable to compare myself to those altruistic moms with boundless energy and enthusiasm for parenting, those who neither undermom nor overmom, when I look at the ledger I've created, I'm just hoping to be closer to Judge Ruth than Dr. Ruth.

twelve

A Million Little Reese's Pieces

My husband takes me to Ojai for the weekend, where we find a little coffeehouse in town and I order a veggie sandwich with pesto and Swiss cheese. I tell myself I'm going to eat only half of it, like an alcoholic tells himself it's just a slice of rum cake and it won't set off a bender and then ends the night with one shoe and forty-seven stitches at County General.

I am just going to eat half the sandwich and wrap up the other half for later. And maybe a few bites of the fruit on the side, because you know, it is Ojai and everything's organic and there must be some nutrients in there the baby sorely needs. Don't want a fetus with scurvy just because I'm trying to keep the eating under control.

And as I'm ordering the sandwich, and planning just to eat half, I'm seriously considering a chai latte, because we're on vacation and it's a vacation chai, and I think I smell nutmeg and what could be as creamy and comforting as a warm spicy beverage on an overcast day? Mommy needs it when she can't even have a glass of wine or a smoke to take the edge off. Everyone knows empty calories take away the empty feelings, or make the thoughts stop skipping like a broken record in my brain: *How much is child care? Is my vagina going to rip when this kid comes out? How exactly do stitches in the vagina feel? Where are we putting the crib? What crib? Are we really supposed to take a parenting class? How much does that C-section thing scar? What is a layette and do I need one? My stomach itches. My stomach itches. My stomach itches.* The doctor advised us to go on a weekend getaway before it was too late to travel, but while my body is only in the second trimester, my mind is in the sixty-third. I actually spend time worrying about my son drinking and driving, which may or may not happen *sixteen years from now.*

And that's where a giant sandwich stops the record skipping with the mollifying power of pesto. Of course, when you use a sandwich to solve a problem, you then have two problems, especially if you're pregnant and running out of stomach real estate.

I feel like someone who has had gastric bypass surgery. My appetite is bottomless, but even half a sandwich makes me feel painfully full and gasping for breath these days.

No matter what I eat these days, even an orange or a handful of nuts, it feels like I have undertaken a massive binge. Whatever is happening to my insides makes me feel both starving and obscenely full almost all of the time. It's weird for your mind to want something your body can't tolerate, to be insatiable and overstuffed, magnetized and repulsed, craving and bursting. I eat the rest of the sandwich before I remember not to.

This leads to a pressure on my diaphragm like someone has glued a thirty-pound lead paperweight to my solar plexus.

No way I'm overeating again, I tell myself, but food amnesia takes hold and by dinner all I can hear is the siren song of homemade corn bread, singing to me from a basket on the table, luring me into dark, carbohydrate-infested waters.

As you may have already deduced, I have an eating disorder, something I've announced hundreds of times after introducing myself at meetings in church basements several times a week as part of a recovery program. This is not a book about addiction, no *Million Little Reese's Pieces*—especially because nothing here is fabricated—but my background of serious body image and food issues does make this weight gain come with a side order of extra disquietude.

After eight years free of crazy eating disorder behaviors, every pound gained makes me question if this is just normal for my particular pregnancy or a little bit of relapsing. As is the tradition in my recovery program, I call a woman every day to check in with her, and she says things sound fine, to take it one day at a time and keep calling her every morning, which I do, but I'm concerned and I never want to go back to how I was.

Look, I wish I had any other kind of addiction, because this one has always seemed the least glamorous, and I'm pretty ashamed at how low a girl can get just because she goes from a size four to a size eight to a size fourteen and back to a size six a couple times a year for twenty years. It wasn't selling my grandmother's wedding ring for crack, but it was demoralizing and isolating, and without help I'm sure I would have ended up eighty pounds or four hundred pounds or dead.

Here's how it looked. As a waitress, I would do things like scarf down the untouched crab cake on a customer's plate while busing it back to the kitchen. As a college student, I would walk two miles in the snow just so I could work out at the gym for hours, which I had to do to burn off the large pizza I would order and eat alone in my apartment. At a temp job once, I was hired to answer phones while the staff went out for a holiday lunch. When they cleared out, I spied a giant vase of M&M's, both plain and peanut. I ate a few handfuls, promised myself I would stop, but couldn't. When the staff returned hours later, their temp was asleep with her head on the desk, candy-colored drool on the sides of her mouth, the vase empty, the phone ringing away. That's how it looked. I know, not exactly *Permanent Midnight*, but a good way to ruin your twenties.

So, you get the idea. Boo hoo, I was a lonely kid who ate candy to keep herself company on the bus and starved to fit in at ballet class and the nuttiness continued into adulthood until I got help.

Hopefully, you can't relate, but maybe you can. In any case, while I have and will continue to make light of my weight gain, it's also a trigger.

I haven't owned a scale in eight years, and I'm not about to buy one now. When you're pregnant, however, the nurse weighs you at every visit, and I have vowed not to let the number scare me into either starving or spinning (on a bike or mentally). It's a medical matter now, more about my ability to carry a baby than carry off a pair of Joe's Jeans. I still go to meetings every week, just to stay connected, and when I introduce myself, I find myself wanting to say, "I'm Teresa, pregnant, not bingeing. I don't have a problem, I have a fetus, so don't bother with the concerned outreach calls but bless you for thinking of me."

While I'm pretty sure my old patterns are in the rearview, so is my size-four body.

When the dust settled on my first trimester, I had gained sixteen pounds.

To put it in perspective, *What to Expect When You're Expecting*, the so-called pregnancy bible reportedly read by 93 percent of pregnant women in America and translated into over forty languages, suggests gaining between two and four pounds in the first trimester. Oops. I saw your two pounds and raised you fourteen.

The author, Heidi Murkoff, delivers this nugget: "Slow and steady doesn't only win the race—it's a winner when it comes to pregnancy weight gain, too."

Heidi and I have broken up a couple of times, but that's because our relationship is kind of intense. I need Heidi when I have scary bleeding—or jammy discharge after my CVS test—and require her hand-holding to be sure everything is normal and not, in fact, a sign of imminent miscarriage. Many a night I've clung to Heidi's comprehensive index (now dog-eared and smeared with Dorito seasoning), looking up spotting, breathing difficulty, hot baths, mood swings, mosquito bites—everything from abscess to zygote. But two to four pounds for the entire first trimester? Is she high? Or just high and mighty?

This is an important, classic and time-tested book, and I acknowledge it is a bible. However, like the Bible, it occasionally says some really fucked-up shit.

"Gradual weight gain also allows for gradual skin stretching (think fewer stretch marks)," adds Heidi, chirpily. And I know a subtle threat when I hear one. Translation in my mind: "Hey, fatty, you keep up the eating if you want an ass full of stretch marks, and don't say I didn't warn you." Still, Heidi is just trying to help and I can't stay mad at her in case I need her stupid index again. In any case, it's not her fault.

But it's not my fault, either. Despite a past filled with treating food like a drug (and, of course, treating drugs like drugs, just never getting hooked), I actually just seem to be eating for a simple, well-adjusted reason: Um, I'm hungry. I'm *huuuuungrry*. And for the first trimester, there was also the queasiness quelled only by crackers and toast, the sudden revulsion toward vegetables, not to mention the quitting smoking.

Now the nausea is subsiding, but the peeing is gaining momentum. There is no such thing as sleeping through the night, because if the hunger doesn't wake me, the hunger to relieve myself will.

This is to be expected. It's almost a pregnancy cliché. Even Heidi will tell you that your bladder is now under pressure, but like most pregnancy symptoms, I'm still surprised by it. It's like, because the pregnancy still seems kind of unreal, the idea that I should expect what other people expect while expecting seems unreal, too. Anyway, every trip to the bathroom reminds me that this pregnancy is sticking, and so while I'm grateful for my crowded bladder, I'm also awakened by it, and if I'm awake, I'm hungry.

I remain ravenously, ridiculously, painfully hungry.

It's the large intestines rubbing together, physical desperation for fried potatoes and eggs kind of hunger you feel when you wake up hungover on a Sunday morning after one too many Jamesons. It's the type of hunger that makes you order a coffee and an orange juice at a diner the morning after and look longingly at your waitress as if to plead, "Seriously, look at me. Get me that juice before you get table four their waffles. This is food and beverage triage, sister, and I'm bleeding out." I want wheels of cheddar, ropes of black licorice and still, strangely, that Guinness beer, which I fantasize about chugging from a frosty stein.

You could probably extrapolate from the above that now, at twenty-one weeks pregnant and just over halfway through, I'm pretty hefty, a weight gain outlier. I've gained twenty-eight pounds so far. According to Heidi, that should pretty much be it for almost the whole pregnancy. Too bad I have four more months to go of important baby growth development time.

Even my ears are fat.

How do I know? Because when I work as a host on a deep cable show that plays on half the screen while the other half scrolls through better programs you could be watching, I use an earpiece (IFB) so the producer can talk to me during the show. About a month ago, it started popping out of my ear. I've used it for years doing live news. As is customary, an audiologist molded the IFB to fit my ear perfectly and no one could figure out why it suddenly kept flying out. It took a new sound guy to point out tactfully that "Sometimes when people change sizes, their ears change shape, too."

I've also outgrown my underpants. I can't bring myself to buy large panties because they remind me of the old days, so I squeeze into medium Victoria's Secret Angel panties just to see how deep and festering a red gash I can acquire from elastic digging into my hip flesh.

One day I catch sight of myself at an outdoor mall, see my reflection in a glass storefront, and can't believe how short my minidress has become because my stomach is pushing the fabric out and consequently up, way up. I have to pop into a Forever 21 to buy a pair of large bright blue fleece shorts. I rip off the tags at the register and pull them on right there.

It's rather uncomfortable adding mass so quickly, because it's something I've done many times before under less delightful circumstances. But my gut, when it isn't busy kicking acid back up into my esophagus, tells me that this isn't a relapse, just my body's way of growing a baby. I may be an outlier, but I'm not a disaster.

I wouldn't trade my worst, sickest, fattest, most bloated pregnant day for not being pregnant at all.

I hope parenting is like that—even days it sucks you would still rather you had done it. And even if it tests the sanity you thought you had before, you don't mind because as far as it stretches you, there is a good chance you will snap back to the basic size and shape of who you were.

It continues to feel surreal that this pregnancy took, that the baby kicks now throughout the day, which is like swallowing a cell phone and taking calls on vibrate. Or sometimes it feels like about a third of the stitch you get in your side when you run too fast. Or maybe popcorn popping.

The fact that it still feels sort of unreal? Unlike the number of pounds I've gained, that is totally, totally normal.

At least that's what Heidi says.

People I Want to Punch:
Don't Touch Me

We pregnant girls are united in what some might call "acquired situational narcissism," but what I prefer to think of as a harmless case of "It's all about us." Who else would even bother pretending to care about nuchal fold measurements or leg cramps?

We need each other. We really do.

That's why I really hate to turn on my own kind . . . but some of them have made my list of people I want to punch.

It seems kind of petty, I know, but I just want to haul off and smack pregnant ladies who get all bent out of shape when people rub their stomachs. You really need to lighten up and get over yourself, two pieces of advice I myself have never been able to take, but which seem very fitting in light of the low level of affront that is actually being done to you. Someone is patting your belly. That's it. It's not like strangers are walking up to you for an ambush fisting. That *would* be rude, and unsanitary. No, they are just grazing your shirt, keeping many layers of fabric, skin, fat, muscle and fascia between their fingers and your future child.

And generally, it is not some belly-molesting evil-doer trying to attack you, but rather a nice, well-meaning person experiencing the magnetic pull of your irresistible, giant bump.

If you don't see why that mesmerizes people, you just don't understand the miracle of childbirth. *C'mon.* Take a step back. A baby grows in your stomach and comes out of your vagina and then goes to nursery school and becomes a full-fledged human being, who may very well create other full-fledged human beings. If you think about it, and I don't suggest you do this high, it's mind-blowing.

I see where you're coming from. I really do. You don't think people should invade your body bubble just because you're pregnant; after all, they wouldn't do this horrible thing to you if you weren't pregnant, wouldn't dream of it. Yes, your body is still your own, absolutely. I just don't quite grasp the near religious fervor that seems to screech, "Don't touch me, because I'm so special that if your grubby hand goes anywhere near my precious child, I'm going to get regular people cooties!"

Do you really need the righteously indignant and

borderline sanctimonious "Hands Off My Bump" maternity T-shirts and others like it that are available online
and also in hell, where ironic maternity T-shirts are very
popular? Talk about literally wearing your aggression
and smugness on your sleeve.

If you want to hear a chorus of pregnant women
shout "Hallelujah," just start going off about strangers
or even relatives touching your stomach, which is why
I really wish I could relate or at least fake agree; I'd love
a chorus behind me and I think it's patently obvious I
need validation like my fetus needs folic acid. I just can't
lie, though. Women who wear those bitter message
T-shirts bother me. Getting riled up about this isn't
nearly as adorably sassy as some women think it is.

I understand pregnancy discomfort and accompa-
nying hormonal moods—I'm sitting here chomping
Tropical Fruit Tums as I type this—but someone feeling
your pregnant stomach really isn't the worst thing that's
ever happened, is it? And the put-upon attitude doesn't
bode well for your maternal future. If someone touching your belly feels invasive, things are *really* going to
get gnarly when the kid invades your space by nursing
on your boob ten times a day, or crying while you're
sleeping, or spitting up on one of your hilarious T-shirts.
Get ready to have your boundaries crossed, because
there are folks who have good reasons to touch your
baby. That's right. Doctors, nurses, midwives, the baby's father, they will all eventually lay their mitts on your
actual young one. The saying goes "It takes a village to

raise a child," not "Everyone in this village better keep their paws off me because I'm more pure than a vat of boiled antibacterial gel in a plastic bubble on Howie Mandel's desk and the villagers are germy, disgusting losers."

It would be nice to think of those of us on the verge of becoming mothers as warm, as cuddly, open creatures who will endeavor to make our babies feel safe and cozy in the world, not as rigid rule makers and enforcers who will crumble the first time some poop lands on our pristine white changing table pad or perhaps works its way into our giraffe-themed nursery throw rug.

I hear tell childbirth is going to be a messy business. Hands will be on us, grabbing or cutting out a kid and possibly helping to shove our nipples into their little mouths.

Hands are going to be on our babies eventually. Yeah, it would be nice if they were free of infectious diseases, but I'm just saying it might be time to loosen the lid on the bottle of "don't touch me."

The whole "Hands Off" movement reminds me of Les Nessman on the sitcom *WKRP in Cincinnati* and the invisible wall he created to delineate his nonexistent office. It was a funny running joke because it pointed to his character's essential immaturity. Grow up. You're pregnant, your stomach is jutting out and people are going to be tempted to reach out and touch it, because that's the human condition. No amount of brassy, finger-wagging, tell-it-to-the-hand antagonism is going to make a wall where there is none.

My *specialty* is whining about nothing, and this annoys even me. So kindly endure the four seconds of bad touch on your stomach or I'll secretly fantasize about coming after your face.

thirteen

Dragging My Names
Through the Mud

One minute, you think naming your son Shane is going to give him a chaps-wearing leg up in life by bestowing on him all the quiet coolness of a 1950s movie cowboy. The next, you're sure naming him Shane will make him the poopy-pants, wheezy outcast who sits out gym class because he forgot his inhaler.

It's a big job, naming a human being.

Girl names are a littler simpler because you can run your nominees through the "attorney/first date" test.

After committing a crime, you don't want to hear, "Hi, I'm your court-appointed attorney, Cinnamon." On the other hand, if I'm fixing you up on a blind date with my cousin, you won't be especially psyched for dinner and a movie with Judith. Basically, choosing a girl name boils down to finding one that doesn't free-associate to either stripper or spinster. She should be fine introducing herself by first name in either a boardroom or the freshman mixer.

When naming a girl, you're just trying to thread that needle, which I think I did with "Harper." In any case, I loved that name and now that I'm having a boy, I can't seem to come up with anything that feels just as right.

For boys, almost every name seems to fall into one of two categories: too boring (John, Robert, William) or too hip (Jasper, Asher, Logan).

Aside from which, our boy will be half Jewish and half Catholic, so his name should suit him in either world. Christopher has always been one of my favorites, but that's not so fun on the *bimah*. I should know about religiously confusing first names, because I'm fairly certain I'm the only Jew named Teresa on the planet. Trust me, no one wants to share a name with a couple of saints when attending Hebrew school with a very elderly teacher who eventually just ends up calling you Rachel, a name you answer to for several years just to save time.

On the other hand, I've always liked having a name that allows me to "pass" as a gentile, because while I love my people, not everyone does, and when I'm in, say, Kentucky reporting a story on the Appalachian poor, it's nice not to have to introduce myself as Shoshana. On that trip, as a matter of fact, I was sitting in a tiny diner eating grits when I overheard this tidbit: "Did you know Jew ladies breastfeed their babies until they're five years old?"

That's when I borrowed my coworker's crucifix for the rest of my stay in Kentucky.

Shoshana might know something about Jew ladies, but Teresa most certainly does not.

All the years asking my parents why they chose such a Catholic name for me, they insisted that it's Hungarian and seemed confounded about why it's a big deal. Now, though, I'm very grateful to be ethnically vague. I'm not going to saddle my child with some unmistakably Jewish name like Chaim (my grandfather) or Irving (two of my uncles), but maybe I don't want to go all New Testament on him either.

Now that I know how hard it is, I can understand why some mothers are so secretive about the names on their short list. First of all, they don't want to finally settle on a name only to have it inevitably slammed. Second, they are afraid of name-napping, a crime I'm flirting with right now. My girlfriend Cassandra is naming her baby Laszlo, and I'm in love with that name. It's different, but not too crazy; it's Hungarian—a tip of the yarmulke to my ancestry; and it alludes to my favorite movie, *Casablanca*, which features the Czech Resistance leader Victor Laszlo.

If you know the movie, you also know there is a character named Major Strasser, who is a major Nazi, which makes it a majorly strange surname when you happen to be a Jew named Teresa.

Still, the connection to *Casablanca* makes the name Laszlo seem even more serendipitous. What's more, it flows well with my husband's consonant-rich Polish name and not many names do. And there's the adorable nickname: Laz. Baby Laz. The more I say it to myself, the more I have to have it.

The ethical and practical questions surrounding name-napping are many. Most people tell me, "They don't own that name. Just take it." However, I plan to see these people and their Laszlo and I don't like knowing that I lacked the creativity to come up with my own darn baby name. Cassandra tells me I can have it, and not in a phony way. She really wouldn't mind if we both have boys named Laszlo, but I would always know in my heart I boosted it. Name-napping may be a victimless crime, but every single time you utter that baby's name, you will be reminded of your own thievery, and anytime the name is praised, you will feel like you have won a Pulitzer Prize for writing you plagiarized.

Running out of time to come up with something original, I ask for suggestions on my blog. Because I haven't settled on a beloved boy name, I'm not worried about strangers crapping on it. In fact, I welcome input.

It turns out, people are passionate about this subject, because we've all either given a name or been given one and anyone who has read *Freakonomics* knows names matter. According to that book's chapter on baby names, it's not that a name influences a child's character, but that the type of parents who choose a particular name may influence a child's character, and thus the destiny of a Destiny has been somewhat preordained. This may be oversimplifying, but as I understand it, if you think the name Destiny is a good idea, you probably think books and nutritious meals are bad ideas, and I apologize to all girls named Destiny, Destinee, Destineigh, Destiknee or Destinay. It's just an example. I'm sure your parents probably did a better job than mine.

As for my son, for the rest of my life, I will have to say his name, scream his name, whisper his name and write his name. Unconsciously, my child will be judged by his name. I've got to really pull something out of my ass here.

I'm thinking James.

You know the trouble with this one: the nickname Jim. Jims seem like nice guys. Jims drive your daughter home from soccer practice without even thinking about molesting her. Jims sell you a used Honda at a fair price. Jims make nifty substitute teachers. I just don't want one. I am told that Jim is an old-school nickname, and that James can now be just James. I have also been told it's becoming a popular girl name. Those greedy little girl parents are taking everything.

I decide to contact a baby name expert, Pamela Redmond Satran (the developer of the addictive site Nameberry.com and the coauthor of *Beyond Ava & Aiden: The Enlightened Guide to Naming Your Baby*). As far as I can tell, she is the baby name maven, and better yet, she seems opinionated. None of this, "The name that feels right to you and your family is the name that's right for you" crap.

Pamela turns out to be a big James fan. As I scribble notes with my phone on speaker and my name expert on blast, she says, "For me, James is really good. And it doesn't have to be Jim, though I actually like Jim. I have a Joe who has never, ever been called Joey, at least by anyone who lived to tell about it. There are lots of Jameses—but not in your neighborhood. Unless they're girls. I really don't think the girls are taking it over, though, not *en masse* outside the hipster ghetto."

Most of the comments on my Web site are pro-James, but several warn me that I will spend a lifetime being the mom who corrects people. "It's *James*." I need to be annoying in other ways.

I'm thinking Mickey.

One word: *Rocky*. You know, "Cut me, Mick." Burgess Meredith, who played Rocky's grizzled old trainer, was iconic as Mickey, and instead of showing my boy *Casablanca*, I can show him another of my favorite films. I also love Denis Leary's sponsor/cousin/former priest, Mickey, from the cable hit *Rescue Me*. Mickey has a solid Irish feel that I love juxtaposed against my husband's super-Polish surname. Mickey loans you money. Mickey plays pool but won't shark you. Mickey knows more than he lets on. Mickey won't sucker punch you, but if you push him too far, he'll break the top off his bottle and threaten you with it just to keep you from acting like a bully. However, does Mickey sound too much like Nicky? And does one have to start with the name Michael to get to Mickey? Will there be lots of Mickey Mouse teasing—you know, M-I-C-K-E-Y? Why? Because your parents chose the wrong name.

After I run this one by my name expert, there is silence on the line for a moment.

"You want to know what I really think? You can't name a kid

Mickey. Yes, there's the mouse, Mickey Rourke, and I dunno, do you really want a son who's the movie sidekick, too good for his own good? Plus, what if he wants to be a bond trader—you're a writer; this could be a good thing—except they won't let him into business school because he's got such an infantile name. I repeat: You can't name a kid Mickey."

This is what happens when you seek advice. Your name gets the axe, or a permanent blemish you can't remove, or a "no" so emphatic you can't pretend you didn't hear it. For every person who loves a name, there is someone who was dumped or fired by someone with that name.

If you've ever loathed a man, you can never again enjoy the smell of that man's cologne. No matter who's wearing it, the scent will make you sick. That's what it's like with names, and maybe my name expert knew some idiot named Mickey and couldn't get the stink off her brain.

My readers bombard me with alternative "M" names like Max, Miles, Milo and Mitchell, all great, but none for me.

I'm thinking Finnegan.

This is the only really quirky name on my short list. Again, I like the mixed ethnicity thing. And the book *Finnegans Wake* took about seventeen years to write, and I like the idea of someone slaving over a book most people can neither read nor understand. And I love the nickname Finn. Is this getting too Aiden/Jaden/Caden? Is Finn trying too hard? Are girls co-opting this one, too?

I'm nervous what Pamela will have to say about this one.

"Finnegan," she repeats. "I actually think Finn is really the better name. Finn McCool is the greatest hero of Irish mythology. Why does everyone think they have to pick Finnegan or Finnian or Finlay and then call their kid Finn? It's not like Jim. Okay, that rant is over. Yes, it is getting too common. It is very easy to like, and that's its problem."

Are there alternatives to Finnegan? I pose the question to the name guru.

"You mean Irish surname-y names? Are you Irish? Do you have any in your family? I do kind of like the Maguire/O'Brien thing, but I think the name's got to be real to pull it off."

Well, my husband is half Irish, so I guess that qualifies us, I tell her, but just barely.

"Here's an Irish name that's totally undiscovered: Piran, patron saint of miners," she adds.

Piran sounds too much like a brand of cookware and now I'm questioning our low level of Irishness.

Plus, there are probably going to be a few Finns in every elementary school class, if the name lady is right, all with parents who thought they were being original. Other Irish names, such as Gavin, Ian, Colm, Dylan, and Rowan, are all either taken by the children of Daniel's Irish relatives or too fancy.

Other quirky names my readers like include Hoagy, Balthazar, Cabot, Miller, Lazare, Kyd, Spider, Stosh, Zeno and Taytum. All are too "Hollywood" for my husband.

I'm still thinking Shane.

The Mister has all but closed the swinging saloon door on this one, but I like it because Shanes are always hot. And he could introduce himself with a joke about how he sounds like a Polish cowboy, and it's nice to have a built-in introductory joke.

My name expert is not ambivalent on this one, either.

"Absolutely no. You're birthing him, not dating him."

Good point. But I hope someone will be dating him, and perhaps the name Shane will help.

A guy named Shane posts on my blog: "My parents named me Shane and I hated it. I remember being two years old and hating my name. I've never stopped hating it. Also, I'm sad to report that not all boys named Shane are attractive."

I'm thinking Edward.

This is racing toward the top for me. Eddie and Ed are cute nicknames. Edward was my grandfather. Sure, he was manic-depressive, but he always had a refrigerator full of Hires root beer and he once made me feel like a genius for getting the word "mauve" in a game of Boggle when I was eight. He told that story until I went to college. Eddie Strasser was my biggest fan.

Is Edward too boring? Will there be too many Edwards in his world? Sometimes my husband test-drives this one by saying "Edward" very sternly to my belly.

I have no idea what Pamela will make of this, the last name on my list. As I'm scrawling notes, I throw this one out at her and hold my breath for a second.

"This is what we wanted to name our second son, now sixteen. We were going to call him Ned. We loved it, and I still do. But our older kids, aged ten and four, said it was a nerd name and they would hate him if we called him Ned, so we didn't do it. And now he thanks us. But I still have regrets and think the *Twilight* Edward has substantially increased the hotness factor. I love this name and definitely think it's the best on your list."

This is a promising endorsement. I wrap up the call and thank her, saying the name Edward to myself over and over as I chew on the moniker and a large pretzel. The only problem is that the name is so strongly linked to my grandfather.

When Grandpa Eddie was in a manic phase, he would bike ride with his grandchildren for miles, take us to the movies, teach us how to sneak in candy we bought beforehand, haul us to the natural history museum and take us to a second movie, all in a single day. On the way home, he would ask my cousins and me what we thought of the film, and if we had nothing to say he would shout, "Stupid! You have to have an opinion. Start talking."

He would often let me sit on his lap while driving and allow me to hold the steering wheel of his beloved powder blue Oldsmobile. The car was striking on the outside, shiny and iridescent like drugstore eye shadow, but suffered numerous intractable engine problems, prompting my grandfather to compare the vehicle to "a Swedish whoooore" (Bronx accent, pronounced like "poor"). "Beautiful on the outside, rotting on the inside."

Because my mom was underwhelmed by the joy of parenthood, my grandparents took me for long stretches during summers and school holidays.

Grandpa Eddie, who called me Butterball when I was chubby, which was most of the time, was about as much fun as a manic grandfather could be. At his funeral, I confided to my brother and cousins that he once pulled me aside and told me that I was his favorite grandchild, because I wasn't quiet and submissive like my female cousins who ran to do dishes after dinner while I pretended I needed to take a shower and hid in the bathroom reading. He loved us all, but had to admit he loved me the most. Turns out, Gramps had similar conversations with all of us, who all thought we were his favorite. Despite this, in my heart, I believe it truly was me, because I was the most broken and had the most to say about the movies we saw.

The downside of being manic-depressive is obviously the depressive part, and when that hit my grandfather a couple times a year, he would take to his bed for weeks at a time, leaning against one of those giant pillows with armrests while staring at the wall.

It was the best of times, it was the most bipolar of times.

As Grandpa Edward's brain chemistry did to his mood, the name pulls me in two directions. There are great memories and painful ones, and maybe I just want a clean slate with my child, a name with no baggage.

Now when I see movies, I not only think about the reviews my grandfather would demand, I not only listen for character names that might work, I also scour the closing credits for baby names. Maybe a gaffer has a name I like. At the bookstore, I stare at spines for authors' first names. I spend hours on baby name Web sites. Every new male I meet is just a name I'm trying on for size. This is my moment, my time to come up with something special but not too special, sentimental but not too closely associated with a specific person, creative but not Apple or Audio Science or Moxie, masculine but not butch, cool but not too easily mocked. Yeah, taking folic acid and not shooting up, those were critical maternal decisions, but this, this feels like the biggy.

I wait. I wait and I hope the baby gives me a clue.

You know how your car stops making the noise the second you take it to the mechanic? That's what my Baby No Name does with his kicking.

The second I put my husband's hand on my stomach, the little guy just stops moving. Today, though, the boy gives a good kick to the palm of my husband's hand for the first time. We're sitting in bed watching *Dateline* as I try breathlessly to get comfortable on seven pillows.

"I felt it. I felt the baby," he says. There it is, our first shared physical experience of our child. I want to get out the camera and videotape it, but grainy footage of happy moments always reminds me of what they show on *Dateline* when someone dies, to reinforce how happy the deceased used to be before being cruelly ripped from this life by a guy they met in a chat room or a drunk driver. I'm too superstitious to tape it, but I try to be still inside myself so I can remember the feeling.

I warn Daniel that I might start crying, which I do.

And it is so sappy and nauseating I'm glad I've already taken a Zantac. I see myself from the outside and think, *Who am I?* I make fun of people who get choked up by things like the miracle of life. I feel superior to people who take this stuff so seriously that they cast plaster molds of their pregnant bellies. I mean, I know it's serious, but these hormones are making me lose my edge, the edge that's probably a fake and carefully constructed defense mechanism to begin with, but it's mine now and I hate to see it crumble.

Struggling to regain it, I stare down at my hand resting on my stomach and blurt, "Quit kicking me, buster!"

"Buster," says my husband. "I like it. Buster."

Until we come up with a real name, Buster it is.

fourteen

Babies 'R' Ripping Us Off

The baby industry says you need to buy everything from nasal aspirators to anal thermometers to layettes and Moses baskets and other possible rip-offs. This triggers my overriding sense that The Man is always trying to gouge me, the same sense that almost made me skip the baby thing in the first place. I didn't want to be "had" and I still don't.

Now big baby stores and ad-driven baby Web sites are trying to convince me I need dozens of products I have never seen and don't understand.

I've never even held a baby and now I have to know whether I really need something called a bouncy seat. Isn't my knee a bouncy seat after an espresso?

These lists overwhelm me and my mind shuts down when forced to confront a world in which bulb syringes, teething toys, colic tablets, bumpers, bassinets, breast pads, burp cloths and tub spout covers play a pivotal role. Most checklists I find for "baby's first year" include upwards of sixty items.

Because I'm superstitious, not to mention paranoid and resentful about perceived consumerist trickery, I figure I'll outsmart the system by simply ignoring it.

I'll wait until the baby is born, see what I actually need, and thus not overbuy—nor tempt fate by filling a nursery with things for a baby that may or may not make it home alive. I know, that sounds dark, but we Jews, after a few thousand years of pain and suffering, really like to manage our expectations. In fact, baby showers were taboo for Jews until pretty recently, and many of us still don't buy so much as a diaper before the baby comes home safely. We avoid broadcasting our good fortune and thus tipping off the evil eye or dark spirits or whoever snatches your baby if you're rude enough to basically brag about it or take it for granted by buying shit. I'm not very religious, but something about this cultural imperative not to get too cocky speaks to me.

Legally I have to buy a car seat, though, which is why I sit down one morning at the kitchen table with my laptop and a toaster waffle and one simple goal: order a car seat online.

Two hours later, I'm sobbing in bed, yesterday's mascara smeared across my pillowcase. I am weeping like Sally Field in *Steel Magnolias'* big funeral scene, yelping in staccato bursts, only no one has died. Nope, I just can't figure out which car seat to buy. Disproportionate emotional response + crying in bed before noon = typical outcome when trying to accomplish difficult task while pregnant.

I consider calling someone, but how can I explain that I've gone full Sally Field because I can't figure out the difference between a Snap-N-Go and a SnugRide?

I had wandered into an online underworld of car seat bases, attachable stroller frames, locking clips, five-point harnesses, boosters and retractable sun canopies. It's like I didn't get the travel warning from the Department of State telling me that going to the Republic of Car Seat by myself was a bad idea. It may look like a peaceful country, but that just makes it all the more dangerous when you don't speak the language.

When I find an expert online to translate, I read this advice: *"Parents often ask which of the many car seats is the best car seat on the market. The truth is, the best car seat is the one that fits your vehicle, your budget, your baby and that you will use properly each time your baby rides in the car."*

Thanks! That's so helpful it requires an ironic exclamation point.

You ever go to therapy, and instead of just having your thoughts and feelings mirrored back to you (*you seem angry at your mother, sounds like work is really frustrating right now*), you really want the shrink to tell you what to do (*break up with him, resign, move out, move in, go back to school, go back to your wife, get a day job*)? Sometimes you need clear direction, you need your GPS to tell you which way to turn, not to ask you which route you think is best for you right now at this juncture of your life. Thanks, baby car seat expert, for telling me I have to look within myself to find the car seat that's right for me, but I wouldn't be going to you for answers if I had any clue so just *give it up.* There must be an overall *best one.* Give me a link, I'll give you my credit card number, and let's do this thing. Just tell me what to do. Please don't make me become a car seat expert when you can save me the trouble by having made yourself one already.

This isn't a life-or-death decision, I try to tell myself as I click around. Oh, wait, I guess it is.

While I can't find anyone to just tell me what to buy, it's no problem finding dire safety warnings about everything from the dangers of buying a recalled model to the likelihood of installing any brand improperly. The implicit communication: If you don't figure it all out, it's on you if the baby flies through the moon roof. *It's on you.*

Worse than the overload, the onslaught of products and the fear-mongering and the confusing plastic parts are the reviews from moms on consumer sites. Wow. These are some opinionated ladies, and they know it all, know every detail about why this travel stroller is too bulky for a trip to Costco and why that one has subpar anchor straps.

Um, I just wanted to have a baby with five seconds to spare before my fertility window slammed shut on my fingers. I didn't want to know about anchor straps.

It's difficult to work up any tolerance for these product-reviewing mothers, who post four-hundred-word treatises on the relative merits of Britax versus Graco. They intimidate me with their superior knowledge of which brands are the most useful, and they rattle me to my very core with their single-minded *momminess*. I don't like how repelled I am by these well-meaning mavens, who just need to share with the world, or at least those on Amazon.com, how the cup holder on the Nautilus 3-in-1 car seat system stroller frame is just too darn narrow for baby's fave sippy cup.

And maybe it's not just about my inability to purchase the ideal base, seat, stroller combination that has me freaked. Maybe it truly is the neighborhood. The enemy doesn't wear a military uniform but a pastel yellow Slurp & Burp nursing cover-up. I'm in my second trimester. I live here now.

For the same reason I resisted baby gear, I was hoping I could avoid buying maternity clothes. I always thought they were a rip-off, but it's futile to resist.

Not buying maternity clothes is like refusing a Xanax on an airplane. Don't be a hero.

A couple of weeks ago, a woman I barely know, but who must now in retrospect be considered a saint, gave me a bunch of hand-me-down maternity clothes. Some fit now, some seem like they'll never fit, but I know they will, and they sit in a stack, waiting.

I never would have purchased this stuff myself, because of my desire to not let the maternity clothing industry squirm its grubby hand into my chubby pocket, but now that I've experienced the magic of roomy camisoles with built-in bras and Empire-waist cotton dresses, I can't look back. The thing about maternity clothes is that they aren't just bigger, like plus-size clothes; they are cut differently, roomier in the right places, and in many cases feature a band of extra-wide, yummy elastic where the waistband of your skirt or jeans would normally be. Anyone who has been pregnant knows this, but it was news to me. Even if you aren't that big, maternity clothes are like Ugg boots for your gut: so comfortable you don't mind looking like you just stepped out of a food court in Lodi clutching a shopping bag from Wet Seal. That's right: You won't look cool—unless you splurge on pricey name-brand maternity denim—but cool is rarely comfortable, and A-line terry-cloth bathing suit cover-ups from Target certainly are. Yes, the maternity stores can jack up prices because they have a captive and nervous audience, but Target, Gap and Old Navy sell some basics that are so cheap you don't feel like a sucker.

And if you hand your maternity clothes over to another pregnant girl when the breeding is all over, you can relish the knowledge that in some small way you are still sticking it to The Man. That's how I justify it, and I plan to pay it forward by passing my black maternity dress pants and every other maternity garment on to the next pregnant chick who is sure she won't need them.

Buying maternity clothes is nowhere near as complicated as buying a car seat; you wear the same size as you did in regular clothes, and if you have a reflective surface, you know whether or not it looks right. You've probably been trying on clothes your entire life, so you know what colors look good on you, you understand the basic idea that pants have two legs and sleeves cover your arms and buttons keep oxford shirts together. This territory isn't so foreign.

Car seat shopping, however, is still breaking my balls.

After hours of searching the Internet and more hours of crying over the fruitlessness of my search, I make the decision that I can never, ever go car seat shopping again. I hand this task off to my husband, and I'm heartened to find that it also makes his head explode. A few days later, we accost a couple on the street with a baby and demand that they give us the make and model of their car seat, which they do, but I think I saw the lady feel around in her purse for her pepper spray. Anyway, that's her problem. We got what we needed, ordered that car seat and had the local fire station install car seat bases in both of our cars.

Comprehending and obtaining this one simple baby product took many days and even more tears. This is an inauspicious beginning for me. How the hell am I supposed to deal with the intricacies of battery-powered, music-playing baby swings? I'm going to have to get a grip on what exactly I need to buy and learn.

Speaking of buying and learning, on top of all the baby and maternity products that are marketed to us pregnant ladies, there are also a bevy of classes, workshops and seminars for sale. Sure, Colonial-era women, or women on the prairie, or women working in a field somewhere, they never needed to take breast-feeding class, swaddling class, infant care seminars, infant CPR or childbirth preparation, but everyone I know seems to be signing up, and that makes me wonder if I should, too.

Our doctor says the infant CPR class is the only one we really need, and I keep thinking how terrible I'll feel if my baby expires because I didn't want to spend a Saturday afternoon in some horribly lit hospital conference room fake-liking other future parents and giving chest compressions to plastic babies.

Maybe I should just find a class and suck it up. Which reminds me, I'm going to have to understand baby bottles, bottle cleaners, bottle warmers and bottle drying racks, which really sucks. Glass bottles are heavy and can break, but plastic bottles contain bisphenol A (BPA), which can, especially when heated, leach into the formula or breast milk and might—or then again might not—be a carcinogen, except for the plastic bottles that are BPA-free; that is, if they're made of nonpolycarbonate plastic like polyethylene or polypropylene.

Figuring out baby products reminds me of doing a crossword puzzle; it makes me feel both stupid and bored.

At least I have a car seat. Anchor straps, nursing bra straps, changing table straps . . . it seems like you're either tethered down or you're free-falling. Only nothing is free. Except the hand-me-downs, of course.

People I Want to Punch: Maternity Models

'm a back sleeper. At least I used to be, until I learned you aren't supposed to sleep on your back after your fourth month of pregnancy, because your huge abdomen chokes off the blood supply to both your heart and the fetus. You're supposed to sleep on your left side, but that feels unnatural to me, and no matter how I situate myself, there is always the sense that I'm suffocating.

This is why I succumb to the pregnancy pillows available online. I buy two, the Snoozer and the Snoogle. (What, the Slumberjack was already trademarked? Couldn't patent Preggy Pillowzzz?) When they arrive, the packages feature photos of pregnant women luxuriously sleeping on these long, noodle-shaped pillows and modeling all the delightful ways one can use them.

It's not that I have anything against these maternity models; it's just that I kind of want to punch them.

For one thing, they seem to be sleeping so peacefully, while I spend my evenings gasping for air and obsessed that my baby isn't getting enough oxygen. While I know they are just models directed to pose in restful tableaus, I hold them responsible for creating what appears to me to be a pregnancy fiction.

For another thing, I'm not even sure if these ladies are even really pregnant. Are they models who just happened to get pregnant and are now trying to get whatever gigs they can until they return to a size zero? Or are they standard models wearing fake stomachs to sell us shit when they aren't even gestating? Who are these women? Hating models is so predictable, and generally, I have nothing but love for beautiful women, but some of these ladies must be fakers. Sure, they have bellies, but their limbs seem suspiciously slender.

And their feet. Let's talk about their tiny, dainty, perfectly manicured feet.

Here's the news: I was a size 9 before the pregnancy and I'm already wearing a 9.5 and inching ever closer to a 10. When this thing is over, I'm pretty sure I'm headed to some kind of special shoe store for ladies with giant feet or transvestites. Maternity models, however, don't have swollen ankles or enlarged feet or even chipped pedicures.

(And by the way, all I want in life is a serious foot rub, but thanks to some mumbo jumbo about acupressure points on the feet and heels triggering early labor, I can't get one unless I show up at the Thai massage place around the corner and try to pass myself off as fat, which seems wrong. This war against foot rubs has worked its way into every corner of the universe. No matter how far off the grid you are, somehow, this information finds you, and now I find myself without anyone who will rub my feet other than my husband, who has already gotten tendonitis in his thumbs.)

The pillow models and their saintly poses and cute bare feet bother me, and so do the models in ads for maternity clothes looking both care- and bloat-free. "Hey, look at me crossing the street in New York City, wearing my smart working-gal separates on my way to a give a PowerPoint presentation looking just like I used to look, only with this cute belly." Or, "Here I am enjoying a summer day with the wind in my hair in this field of lavender wearing a stylish white maternity sundress and not at all worried that there isn't a bathroom for miles." Or, "Hey, buy this polka-dot maternity bathing suit and suddenly, like me, you will no longer be mopping sweat from between your boobs and overheating like a Chevy Vega in Khartoum." I know all models are hired to create illusions, and usually I'm okay with that, but not right now.

My skin has finally cleared up, but that doesn't mean I can't water my grudge garden when it comes to porcelain-skinned "pregnant" women hawking pregnancy wares from skin cream to nursing bras with their perfectly rosy complexions.

I get so jealous that I even want to punch cartoon drawings of pregnant women, like the one on the cover of a book someone gave me about finding mom bargains in Los Angeles. This cover girl may be a cartoon, but with her hip outfit, high ponytail, flowing scarf, giant sunglasses and overflowing cobalt bag, she is trotting around ready to take the world of maternity and motherhood by storm, and looking effortlessly chic doing it. She does not exist, which will pose a problem when it comes to punching her, but the least I can do is cultivate a low-grade resentment that I will never be as fashionable and breezy as she is.

Being pissed off because models are not only genetically gifted but also Photoshopped isn't something I endorse. I get that pretty people with airbrushed flaws make us want to buy stuff, and that's what makes the world go round. However, while I understand that not all pregnant women have estrogen surge–induced acne and binge-induced upper arm fat, most of us are struggling with physical changes and it would be nice if maternity models didn't always look so flawless and joyful.

The changes aren't permanent, at least I hope they aren't, so I'm trying to keep my chins up about it, but maternity models, I'd still like to punch you in yours.

fifteen

Pregnancy Sex Doesn't Suck, but Maybe You Should

A girl bragging about her great sex life is beyond annoying.
I'm making an icky face just thinking about it, recalling a friend I once had who always sat on her boyfriend's lap in public, even at small gatherings, and insisted on showing me little movies of his "amazing" penis she took on her cell phone. *That's nice. Don't ever show me that again.* What I wanted to say was that couples who rub their seemingly superior sexual devotion and compatibility in your face are almost always the ones who are about to break up in spectacular fashion. Case in point: That girl with the cell phone video of her boyfriend's wang, she found out he was cheating on her and he tried to win her back by confiding about his troubled childhood, including a long-standing sexual relationship with his sister. I'm not saying all sex braggers are incest-surviving sexual exhibitionists working out issues, but there's usually a story.

Remember Angelina Jolie wearing Billy Bob's blood in a vial around her neck and making out on the red carpet while insinuating that they had just had sex in their limo? Or "made love," as they probably put it? You knew it was over.

Pam Anderson tattoos Tommy's name on her person, and it isn't long before she's having to change "Tommy" to "Mommy," which seems kind of sweet in light of my current condition, but I must say the success rate of gals who tattoo wedding rings on their fingers seems frightfully low.

What, am I British all of a sudden? Not just the fancy Anglican adjective, but also the prudishness.

It's a beautiful thing when a man and a woman have sexual chemistry. I just don't want to hear about it, and I notice that when I do, it usually seems like a message is being crammed down my throat about what's being crammed down her throat.

So back to my awesome pregnancy sex and how I'm going to tell you about it.

I do this only as a public service, and I feel justified because most of what you hear about pregnancy sex is negative, and this might alter your expectations, or give you something to look forward to. Or just gross you out, for which I apologize. Besides, I think my surfeit of unfortunate pregnancy symptoms buys me a little leeway here.

Most women I know don't care for pregnancy sex. They feel big, they feel queasy, they can't find a comfortable position, and in some cases it creeps out their husbands to think of their penis going anywhere near their future child. For many, there is something psychological to be gotten over when it comes to pregnancy sex.

I was prepared to feel the stereotypical aversion, so I am shocked and kind of confused about the reality of second-trimester sex for me: It's good. It's really, *really* good.

I don't mean because of the deep soul connection of two people who are creating a human life and preparing to share the mystical voyage of parenthood. No. I mean, all of that can't hurt, but that's not what I'm talking about. I'm talking about the physical. The "happy ending" is just *happier*, as if the purely physical part of the sexual pleasure equation has increased by orders of magnitude. At my last checkup, I even asked the doctor about it, just to make sure my girl parts weren't going haywire. He said increased blood flow to the pelvic region and hormonal changes can make some women extra orgasmic, a word I vow never to use again, but look, there's such a dramatic upturn in sensation that it demands mentioning, even if it makes me sound like the horny upstairs neighbor on *Three's Company*. I don't relish coming off like I'm toasting the sexual revolution over at the Regal Beagle with Jack and Larry, but there is no other way to put it.

At least for me, the physiological effects of carrying a child are making me feel sexy, cankles and all.

While the fog of my cognitively impaired baby brain has reduced my ability to do just about everything, it's really helpful to be stupid sometimes, especially when it comes to sex. That ten minutes it usually takes my mind to wind down, stop making to-do lists and just focus on foreplay, that ten minutes when my brain is like a thought blender set on mince, that is gone. I can't keep track of things, I lock myself out in my pajamas from time to time and I regularly find myself in a state I would describe as addled, buzzed and a little bit blank—in other words, a perfect way for a chronic overthinker to enjoy something as basic as human touch. Oh, no, I grossed myself out again.

There's another thing.

I was on the pill for about five thousand years, and it strikes me that maybe those pharmaceutical hormones, while helping keep my cramps and flow under control, were messing with my sexual mojo. Now, I'm Yaz free, with no worries about birth control or even fertility. As a matter of fact, this is the first time in my life I've had sex without worrying about getting pregnant or not getting pregnant. Throw in a couple extra pints of blood floating around, chemical changes, ultrasensitive but not yet painfully enlarged boobs, and a frontal lobe that's on pause, and you have a recipe for the best sex of your life. Or it could just be an awkward mess that skeeves you out. If so, I'm sorry.

Pregnancy sex is also an opportunity to learn something about men that you may have heard, but never truly believed. All of the little physical so-called imperfections that disturb you, the ingrown hair, or botched eyebrow waxing, or mismatched bra and panties, most men don't notice, and if they do, they don't care.

I once asked a male friend, "What is your type?" He gave me an answer that stuck with me.

"The type who will agree to have sex with me."

Thus, when you are puffing up, with a linea nigra (that hyperpigmented vertical line going from your belly button to your pubic bone), when you have greasy skin, when you are so huge you can no longer even see your own vagina, you will still be your man's type, if you agree to have sex with him. He doesn't care about the elastic giving way on your tap pants or even your lack of pruning down there.

If he is one of those guys who doesn't want to have sex with you because your body looks different now, or because you are about to become the mother of his child, there is probably something wrong with him. Maybe a scarring religious background or some kind of down low gayness, which certainly isn't "wrong" wrong, but it's wrong if you were hoping he was straight.

That is overly judgmental and simplistic. I'm just trying to take the focus away from my bragging about my great pregnancy sex.

I totally get it if you're one of these women who is just too dis-tracted of mind or tender of body to bother with intercourse while gestating a baby. I'm not over here all "Look at me! I'm a goddess of sexual satisfaction." If not for my fluke-y increase in responsiveness, I'm sure I'd be right there with you.

There is, however, one more thing to consider. While the science may be shaky on this, I stumbled across some information about pregnancy sex that doesn't suck, but suggests that you do. I will try to be delicate about this, but let me pass along my two-bit research and tell you how, in a roundabout way, Dr. Quinn, Medicine Woman, was responsible for prescribing not just oral, but specifically perform-ing oral sex and swallowing.

One of my favorite pregnancy hobbies continues to be obsessively researching dangerous pregnancy-related conditions. I know, I know, I could knit, but that would be relaxing, whereas this is more congru-ent with my other top pastimes, which include rehearsing painful conversations I'm going to have in the future and raking over ones I've had in the past. Anyway, after I interview the actress Jane Seymour for my talk show on deep cable (that's right, not only Dr. Quinn but an early Bond girl, mother of six, and one of the most gorgeous and forthcoming moms I have met), I have to look up preeclampsia. She said she got it during one of her pregnancies, and I figured I needed a new worry charm for my shiny bracelet of maternal concerns.

(She also whispered "get an epidural," which I take seriously, be-cause her dad was an ob-gyn. Plus, did I mention she has six kids?)

First, I go home and find a concise description of preeclampsia on the Mayo Clinic's Web site: "A condition of pregnancy marked by high blood pressure and excess protein in your urine after 20 weeks of pregnancy."

This merits a trip to Wikipedia, where I find all sorts of links to academic papers on the subject, and buried therein the suggestion that pregnant women should not only give oral sex but make sure to swallow the semen of their baby's daddy.

After I do some digesting about ingesting, I have to stand up from my desk chair and say to no one in particular, "Really?" If I've heard about a new mother eating her own placenta in a panini to ward off depression, or chanting "I and my baby are experiencing immense joy and happiness" for ten minutes after doing Kundalini yoga, if I've scoured mommy blogs and parenting sites for every possible detail about a healthy pregnancy, how have I missed this gem?

Maybe small-scale studies from Dutch researchers in obscure medical journals don't find a wide audience. Or maybe penises need a new publicist.

I'm no doctor, just a pregnant lady with an Internet connection, so maybe I'm horribly confused, but it sounds like if you're thinking about conceiving, or certainly if you are already pregnant, there is some pretty convincing evidence that instead of just swallowing, say, folic acid, you might want to swallow something else. Here is what I found excerpted online, from the *Journal of Reproductive Immunology*: "The epidemiological indication that oral sex and swallowing sperm might have a protective effect in the occurrence of preeclampsia, fits with the concept that exposure to paternal antigens prior to gestation has a beneficial effect towards normal pregnancies."

That is from a paper by a team of Dutch researchers with the catchy title "Correlation between oral sex and a low incidence of preeclampsia: a role for soluble HLA in seminal fluid?" Or as it should be subtitled, "Semen is your friend."

Basically, the research says you need to be able to tolerate your baby's foreign, paternal DNA, need to get your body accustomed to the stuff, need to cozy up to some daddy double helix for a while so your body doesn't reject it.

I could not make this up. This study and several other jauntily titled articles from dense publications on obstetrics and immunology suggest that while any exposure to a partner's semen is good, gastrointestinal absorption may be the best. *Gastrointestinal absorption of semen.* I know.

As far as I can tell, not only should you be having lots of oral sex with the father of your baby—even up to a year before conceiving—you should also make sure to ingest his seminal fluid. Sure, the researchers say frequent intercourse is good, too, but oral is better because it promotes that superior gastrointestinal absorption.

For the man in your life, this news should not be hard to swallow. Even if that joke is.

I just can't figure out why the whole "blue balls" thing has gotten so much traction with men, but they haven't gotten ahold of this medical morsel. Sure, the studies were small and who knows if they were ever replicated, but guys didn't have much to hang their hats on with blue balls, and yet that one has been around forever, used to persuade women that having a prolonged hard-on without orgasm carried the grave danger of some kind of toxic testicular congestion. Or at least that's how it was explained to me at Jewish summer camp.

While I'm sure it's uncomfortable, even back in the day I was dubious about the dire medical consequences of not "finishing." This swallowing stuff, though, I'm telling you, it kind of makes sense.

Now, to be fair, the Dutch researchers do warn that with a new partner, condoms should be used to prevent sexually transmitted diseases. However, they insist, a certain period of sperm exposure within a stable relationship, when pregnancy is aimed for, is associated with partial protection against the dreaded preeclampsia.

Again, I'm obviously not a scientist, so to conclude, I will fall back on the medical opinion I always have about things that are either Suzanne Somers-y or reeking of placebo-ness, but obviously benign: It can't hurt, right? At the very least, your baby will have a happy, relaxed father and parents who are intimate.

You're welcome, dads.

sixteen

Hey, Other Pregnant Ladies:
Look My Way

Everyone is so nice to you when you're pregnant. Everyone, that is, except other pregnant women.

Listen, expecting girls, all I want to do is talk to you, find out how many weeks pregnant you are and maybe talk some shop—you know, where you're delivering, what you take for heartburn, what you think of cord blood banking and the new iPhone app that times contractions. I just want to be friends, Pregnant Strangers.

However, it seems you gestational types aren't really feeling me.

At first, I wanted to make sure you knew that I wasn't just carrying my weight in a very unfortunate manner, that I was really pregnant rather than just someone who binged on scones and cans of frosting. I would rub my stomach in the gingerly way only pregnant women do, try to catch your eye, but no dice. To be honest, I've been a social disaster most of my life, so I'm not unfamiliar with the sensation of being snubbed—I just can't figure out why this dismissal is so pronounced.

I'm always hoping we're going to see each other and, you know, have a moment. I mean, if we ran into each other carrying the same L.L. Bean tote bag, we would probably at least chuckle and say, "Nice purse." A richly hued and hilarious interaction it would not be, but a human connection, yes.

If I were walking a beagle and so were you, wouldn't we stop and have a chat about our beagles? Arguably, an entire friendship could spring forth from this one shared characteristic. If we were both wearing Phillies hats, or driving Mini Coopers, or reading *Eat, Pray, Love* at the Coffee Bean, there would likely be warm dealings, but both heading into childbirth (big deal) and motherhood (biggest deal ever) and nada. *Nada?*

Important point: This pregnant girl snubbing only pertains to complete strangers.

I need some home girls. Sometimes I'm euphoric and sometimes I'm sweating pit stains through my muumuu. I have vivid dreams about epidurals and blinding surgical lights. When you're lost on the subway in a foreign country, you look for anyone else who speaks your language, because either they can help you or you can be lost together.

You pregnant ladies who walk right by me on the sidewalk and turn away like I'm about to make you sign a petition about saving marine life, I know you can relate.

So I can only imagine there is some sort of animal kingdom thing at play here.

Maybe this is insane, but it's almost like I represent a threat, another mother bear that might somehow compromise your safety or shrink your available resources. Is there something evolutionary going on, as in, *That lady better not get more shelter, berries, attention, or protection from strong males in the tribe?*

Alternatively, this could be peculiar to the Hollywood area, where

I live and write in various coffee shops and drop off dry cleaning and wander. I'm told the Midwest, the South, heck, even the Valley—those are great places for pregnant bonding.

Or, both of these theories could be bogus. In the classic horror movie *When a Stranger Calls*, the most chilling scene is when cops tell the terrorized babysitter, "The call is coming from inside the house." There is a decent chance that this call is coming from inside my own haunted mind. Either I am unknowingly giving off a frosty vibe that turns off the strange women I'm hoping to befriend or I'm reading into this parade of pregnant girls some animosity that doesn't exist.

Like I said, my social skills have never been great.

What if, with our giant bellies and off-kilter walks and vulnerable demeanors, we are simply used to being the center of attention, and we unconsciously despise sharing the spotlight?

In any case, this could all be solved with an ice-breaking secret handshake. Or if that's too intimate, maybe we just throw up a sign, one finger per trimester, sideways, OG-style, and know for a sly, passing moment that we're in the same crew.

One afternoon, I'm meeting one of my girlfriends for a movie, standing outside the theater. There is one other woman waiting there, who is also visibly pregnant. I'm pretty sure we're even wearing the same black Gap maternity leggings. I try to make eye contact, but she looks away.

As people walk in and out of the movie theater, they notice us, a matched set, standing a few feet apart, and I can swear they are thinking, "Maybe you two should chat." But we don't. It's a bizarre standoff, and when my pregnant friend Christy arrives, there are three of us and I'm sure this lady is going to make contact, maybe joke about how between the three of us, there are six trimesters. Or maybe she'll say something about how we'll all be spending the entire movie running to the bathroom, or eating buckets of popcorn. At the very least, can this woman eke out a "When are you guys due?"

No.

This is why I'm thankful I've latched onto my new crew. I have now made three new friends, simply because we are all pregnant at the same time. Hanging out with them feels both right and comfortable.

Christy is a friend of my friend Ben. Both are movie critics. She is a month behind me, heard about me from Ben, asked for my number and invited me out on a blind date for coffee, where we proceeded to talk for hours about vaginal tearing and finding day care. When you're pregnant, you think almost exclusively about your condition, and desperately want to talk to other people who are right there with you, find out what's on their registries or how much alcohol their doctor allows. You'll want to commiserate about the time-consuming gestational diabetes test that involves drinking a cup of syrupy cola-type stuff and waiting an hour before having your blood drawn. You'll want to compare pounds gained and appointments forgotten due to "baby brain." You'll get over any social phobias you may have had just to have someone to text about every doctor visit and symptom.

When my radio show went off the air, a magazine writer who had been a guest a few times wrote me to say he was sorry we got canceled, and that his wife was also pregnant.

"Really? Can I have her e-mail?" I wrote back. And that's how I befriend Cassandra, who is months ahead of me, close to delivering.

Like me, she was never baby crazy, but she seems way more on top of things than I am. She sends me a list of birth doulas. She plans on using cloth diapers and having her placenta cooked and turned into tablets to stave off postpartum depression. I respect her hippie ways, and the fact that she has dedicated herself to learning about the foreign world of baby birthing while I sit around paralyzed like a pregnant fly in hardening amber. Also, she hates being pregnant and has gained fifty pounds, which I am on pace to do, and she makes me feel better about the fact that not every day is joyful or certain. There are moments I ask myself, "What have I gotten myself into?" and that's a sentiment you can only share with other pregnant girls.

Jen, who has also done a few tours of duty hosting on basic cable, is a woman I met through Christy. She gets bonus points for also having a troubled relationship with her mom and being a few months older than I am.

Before being pregnant, I didn't even know these women, and now I'm pretty sure I can't go a day without contacting at least one of them.

At camp, in college, at my first newspaper job, at my first television writing job, I always fell in with a small, tight group and thought, "I love these people, and we'll all be friends for life." Now I'm lucky if I recognize their photos when they contact me on Facebook. The point is, going from city to city and job to job, I tend to get very close to people quickly and just as quickly move on, but in this case, we'll all be moms together. We'll still need each other. And that's a bond that has to last.

Christy, Jen and I go to lunch together in Burbank one afternoon. The host gives us a special booth in the back with lots of room for our giant stomachs. We discuss baby names and stretch mark creams. It's dark in that back room and cozy and I never want to leave there, just want to eat melted cheese off French onion soup and discuss baby stuff into the night in our dim womb of a booth. Plus, it's pretty hard for me to get my unwieldy body back out, so the desire to stay there is both emotional and practical.

It's a tale of two types of pregnant girls, the ones who are on your team and the others, on the visiting team, who stink eye you.

What's amazing is that the rest of the world, they kiss your ass. The cashier at the grocery store smiles at you extra wide, the saleslady at the maternity store asks if you need some water, the receptionist at the chiropractor asks why you didn't wear a sweater on a cold day.

This is, by far, the best thing about being pregnant.

Since I was little, I wanted the gold star, wanted to win the spelling bee, win at kick ball, win awards and otherwise prove myself in ways that were public and indisputable.

This is very simple, as far as psychological analyses go. My stepmother spent fifteen straight years convincing everyone that I was a chubby, devious, sloppy, rude, outcast loser who would never amount to anything. I just wanted to prove her wrong, and even though she's been in the ground for five years now—ground I would tap dance on in a red dress if that wasn't just a figure of speech and she wasn't, in fact, cremated—I can't stop trying to rub her cold, dead nose in her wrongness about me. It's not a great raison d'être, having to excel in the world because my evil step-monster said I couldn't. It's exhausting and often results in failures feeling bigger than they are, and achievements causing a brief high that fades, leaving nothing but a gaping hunger for shinier gold stars.

For the first time, I can let go of all my trying.

The world is opening doors for me and holding my bags and rubbing my shoulders not because of anything I accomplished in my career but simply because I'm smack in the middle of this run-of-the-mill human rite of passage that makes people want to take care of you. The relief is like a Tums to my frontal lobe. I can relax and the world won't forget me.

Biology has taken over. The attention I once chased was contingent on my being excellent, and that gave me everything from writer's block to crippling stage fright. On my way to speak to two hundred people at a university one Friday night, I got out of a moving car because I was so petrified of performing. I spent twenty minutes on the side of the road reciting affirmations from a book called *Stop Obsessing* before I could get back in the car. When I used to do live hits for a national news show, I would shake so badly it was hard to hold the mic still while covering a parade or interviewing Brad Pitt. Now, my body is doing something cool without my mind's help, and everywhere I go the belly is buying me 27 percent more human kindness. Despite the worsening discomfort, this makes me want to be pregnant forever.

The effect is so pronounced that being in my car, where other drivers can't see that I'm pregnant, is confusing.

When a car doesn't let me merge, I find myself momentarily shocked at not being given the right of way. I start to feel like I should be allowed my own siren, to snap on top of my car so I can speed home when I have to pee, which is all the time. Some malls have a few parking spots designated for "expecting moms," which makes me feel like I should have my own space everywhere I go, because my feet are swollen and, c'mon, it's *me*, with child. I should be allowed to speed, go through stop signs, park when there's street cleaning, drive in the carpool lane and forget to signal. Everyone should clear out when I'm trying to exit the clogged parking lot at Trader Joe's. I'm making a baby, and everyone should make a big deal out of it, and take care of me, and know just by looking at my car that there's precious cargo inside and thus the rules, like my pants, should have plenty of give. It's a peculiar mix of entitlement and fragility.

I wonder if other women feel like this when they're in their cars, if they feel weak and protective and huge and hulking all at the same time.

That's why we need each other, to make sure we aren't insane. Sure, women have been doing this forever, but that doesn't matter at all when you're a rookie. When you're standing at the plate facing a ninety-mile-an-hour pitch in front of a packed stadium, it doesn't matter at all that every big leaguer before you has been there. That fastball is still coming at you, and the stakes are painfully high. Even if your dugout is just a booth at a restaurant in Burbank littered with breadstick crumbs, you've been drafted, and you better make some friends on the team. At the moment of truth you're out there alone, but before you step up to the plate, you can get some scouting reports, a pinch of chewing tobacco and an encouraging pat on the butt. They may not help you get on base, but they know exactly how the butter-flies feel.

seventeen

A Cut Above (the Anus)

L et me throw these two words at you: fecal incontinence.
     Now that I'm six months pregnant, I have finally gotten
around to taking a break from worrying about what kind of mother
I'm going to be in order to get to the urgent business of stone-cold
panicking about how this Buster kid is getting out of me, and what
damage he might do as he leaves. At my last doctor visit, we had the
episiotomy talk, and now I can't stop thinking about the potential
slicing of my privates, or the uncontrolled tearing, or the aforementioned fecal freaking incontinence, which happens to some women
after childbirth.

According to Rod Stewart, "the first cut is the deepest," but I
think it's safe to say any cut that might lead to bowel leakage is the
deepest, at least emotionally and spiritually.

First- and second-trimester concerns now seem almost quaint in
their solvability. Nauseous? Enjoy some ginger chews and pop some
B_{12}. Leg cramps? Stretch your calves before bed and eat a banana.
Your baby's head is too big to exit your vagina? Slice open the area

between your anus and vulva, stitch it back up, and hope you don't end up with the inability to control the seepage of gas and stools from your bowels due to a torn sphincter.

Perhaps I was intentionally fuzzy on the episiotomy thing. I wasn't ready to know about my perineum (or "taint," as it is often called, because it 'taint your vagina and 'taint your anus). Call it squeamishness, or immaturity, or just plain intentional ignorance.

That is, until my doctor tells me that he is a big fan of cutting, that most women will tear, and if you do a preemptive cut, you can control the severity and direction, keeping the tear away from the bad place. Fecal incontinence and severe, lingering sexual pain averted.

Sounds reasonable to my husband and me, until we go home and consult a few pregnancy books and Web sites, most of which suggest that cutting is old school, and that perineum massage during labor can help the vaginal opening stretch, leading to just a small tear or no tear at all. Friends who have had babies are all over the place, some insisting, like my doctor, that cutting saves you from a jagged tear, others saying a rip is more natural and heals more easily.

I'm in labial limbo—okay, not precisely, but alliteration is so seductive. I have no idea which is best, and I assume it depends on you, your baby, and your labor, but I guess you probably want a doctor who hopes for a neat little tear but makes a cut if need be.

At times, I feel guilty for making such a big deal out of this cut/tear thing when I'm bringing a person into the world. Why should I care so much about my little old vagina and anus? That's when I come to my senses. This is a big deal. *Fecal incontinence hangs in the balance.*

When I found out I was pregnant, it took me by surprise, because of my plan for a lengthy, draining bout of infertility. So I hadn't put much thought into choosing a doctor, and in fact, I just picked a guy my makeup artist recommended because he had an open appointment and she said he gives a heck of a Pap smear. I didn't interview him about his philosophies on childbirth, nor did I ask any of the questions that now seem pertinent—his thoughts on C-sections or epidurals, for example. I didn't know any mothers who recommended him. For some reason, I didn't want to be the woman who goes around with a clipboard auditioning doctors. When I started to meet other pregnant ladies, however, I realized this was a blunder, and that I really didn't know much at all about the guy who was going to deliver my child. And now that we've been together awhile, shared some good news and fun sonograms together, it seems hard to break up and start all over with a new ob-gyn.

My plan is to take the path of least resistance, and hope my vagina does likewise.

When it comes time to choose a doula, an assistant who provides nonmedical support during labor, I'm more careful. Okay, I interview one lady and hire her, but I love her instantly and she isn't as hard-core on the no pain meds front as others might be. And I like her name: Margie. Who doesn't want a Margie around when they're dilating? Because Margie has been around the birthing business for years, I ask what she thinks of my doctor, who seems nice enough other than telling me, "You only get two questions per visit," and of course his dubious love affair with the preemptive episiotomy.

Margie, without blinking, says, "Oh, the Vagina Butcher? That's what we call him. I mean, it's up to you."

And I know I have to get out. Had I bothered to do any digging, I would have known sooner that my doctor has a nickname in the doula community. He butchers vaginas, apparently. So, I do the honorable thing and have my husband call and say we're moving to another city. Daniel gets my medical records faxed to him so there is no awkward good-bye and I'm now in the care of a new doctor, a mother of two with a nice practice in Glendale. The new doctor is someone Margie knows, has worked with before and trusts. That's good enough for me. There are a few very popular and beloved doctors in Los Angeles and sometimes I get doctor envy for not having someone fancy or famous, but at least my new doc only plans to cut my vag if it's absolutely necessary.

Don't go Googling this topic, because while you will find delightful tales of intact girl parts, you will just as surely find horribly misspelled, sad, angry postings about "fourth degree" tears, leaking, burning and bleeding that you can't ever un-read. The Internet is the Heidi Montag to my Lauren Conrad. That's right, we're frenemies. The Web is my friend when I find a posting by someone sane who has survived childbirth without anal stress incontinence, but it's my enemy when I get sucked into some rambling, under-punctuated story about a years-long recovery from an epic laceration.

I comfort myself with the notion that just as boots are made for walking and kidneys are made for filtering, vaginas are made for stretching. I should be fine. Sometimes, this is obvious, and other times, it 'taint.

People I Want to Punch:
So in Love with Big Boobs

know having "big balls" is prized, at least metaphorically, but guys, if you happen to be reading this pregnancy book, imagine if your balls were three times their normal size, swollen, sensitive, hanging heavy and splaying uncomfortably across your thighs. Big, giant balls would get in your way, as awesome as they sound.

Guys may want brass balls, or balls of steel, they may even want to go balls to the wall, but big balls? I would think twice now that I know how big boobs feel.

All the people who relish big boobs, who comment on how much I must love the new rack, sometimes I want to punch you.

I was an A cup and now I'm busting out of a C. And it's not all that. One afternoon, I'm sitting having coffee with a friend when the front clasp of my bra comes undone, apropos of nothing, and I just bust out of my brand-new Spanx bra. Maybe it was caused by the dangerous mixture of a robust inhale with a moment of slight slouching. Basically, I'm sitting stock-still inadvertently flashing the place (probably should have buttoned those top few buttons on my oxford) before I process what has happened. I don't blame the bra, but my boobs are growing so fast they are actually testing the tensile strength of Spanx.

This is supposed to be one of the best things about being pregnant, but I didn't mind my old A cups. These new boobs are tender and unwieldy. It's hard to sleep without rolling over and pinching one of them. Sometimes I can actually feel growing pains in one or the other, like when my mind wanders during a boring movie (thanks, *Angels and Demons*, for giving me 138 minutes to notice the stinging, aching feeling of my breasts inching toward a D cup).

I keep trying to wear the little bralette things I used to wear—you know, no underwire, no hooks; you just slip them over your head and they look sweet and girlie—but now they feel suffocating, like something Joan of Arc would have worn to bind herself down and pass as male. Either Joan of Arc or Yentl. Or Brandon Teena.

When people comment on my emergent boobs and how thrilled I must be, they are essentially telling me that my regular size, to which I assume I will return, is inferior. Well, oddly enough, being flat-chested is one of the only things about my appearance that I don't mind, which is strange considering I live in Los Angeles and should be on my third set of implants by now.

Whereas I once clung to my flat status as making me stand out in a world of curvy women, now I'm a C, which is to say, average, and in my case, painfully average. No more not needing a bra, or even taking for granted that I will stay in one. No more pain-free jogs on the treadmill. No more looking athletic in a men's oxford. It's a new world, and in this new world, I have to pay attention to "support" and coverage and cleavage.

I'm not saying I'm all offended that our culture prefers giant-breasted women; it's just that I had carved this out as my one area of beauty confidence and now I must humor all of you joking about how my husband must be psyched and how much I'm going to be sad when these breasts deflate.

This is physically uncomfortable and it doesn't make me feel more womanly or more attractive, so when I have to go along with all of you saying how much fun it is to have boobs now, I want to punch you a little bit. Just please, if you have to punch me back, not in the chest. Thank you.

eighteen

Babymoon in Vegas:
Bet on a Crisis

On the way to Vegas, things start to go wrong, as they so often do, at the Mad Greek.

Within a couple of hours, I will be trying to locate the nearest hospital, but now I'm just waiting for the beefy leather-skinned guy in front of me to stop yelling at the clerk about his $3, and how it was her mistake, and how he's going to file a claim with the state. Behind me, a man eats sullenly at a booth with his well-behaved toddler, who silently chews one fry after another.

The roadside diner smells of coconut sunscreen, with base notes of diesel and feta.

I had begged my husband to take me to Vegas, because I was doing what they call in recovery programs "pulling a geographic." As in, *If I just leave Colorado, I won't wake up with festering facial sores and paranoia, because I'm not really a meth addict. I just need to move to Boston.* Instead of going on a normal "babymoon" to, say, temperate San Diego, I decide that in Vegas I'll be the old me.

Baker, California, is right off the I-15. I've broken down here many times. In the past, it was just my car overheating, or my psyche decompressing from a weekend with my mom and her wall of bird-themed paintings and her obsessive studying of restaurant menus and her autistic tuning out. This time, however, it's my body. I'm twenty-nine weeks pregnant, it's 110 degrees, I have no business being at the Mad Greek no matter how much I love their greasy pita bread and fresh strawberry shakes, no matter how much I think the me that will show up in Vegas for a last hurrah won't look like she's in her sixth trimester, or have trouble breathing, or be sure she's washed up in show business or be concerned her baby won't be healthy or his life won't be perfect.

Ojai in the second trimester was one thing, but the third trimester is no time to head into a desert, much less toward Vegas, a city filled with smoke-choked casinos, frat guys who shove you blithely on elevators, free booze you can't drink, mile-long walks to everything, hooker-strippers whose frosted hair and legginess are an attack on your swollen feet and maternity maxi-dress.

Unfortunately, wherever you go, you take yourself with you, which is another one of the annoyingly true bumper-sticker slogans they tell addicts. The same holds for pregnancy, and the crappy mood that has come with it for the last couple of weeks, and the not working much anymore and the visions of myself rocking a baby with spit-up on my shoulder staring blankly at a newborn and asking myself, "Is this how I'm supposed to feel?"

In Vegas, or I should say en route to Vegas, I am still big and un-comfortable and scared with a tinge of pre-postpartum. Only on I-15, I don't drink any water because I'm nervous about having to pee.

At the Mad Greek, I order an omelet. When the cashier asks me what kind of toast I want, I hesitate, ask what they have. I mumble "wheat," and look backward at my husband, as if to ask, "Do I really want wheat bread toast? Will that taste good to me? Would I prefer rye? Who am I?"

He snaps, "Yes. Wheat. Good." Only I would know he's snapping, because he's a subtle snapper. My husband has a very long fuse and almost never loses his temper, but when you're this pregnant, you can't sustain even a small snap.

I slide into a booth as he waits for our order, sip on my fountain drink, eye the kid eating his fries. Feel a kinship with the little dude in his denim overalls, because we both seem lost and like we need our mommies.

My husband returns with our food, which we both just stare at until I tell him I didn't like him snapping at me, and he apologizes, and admits he has spent the last two hours regarding the temperature gauge, worried he was going to break down on the side of the road with his pregnant wife. He's been worried about lots of things, he admits: being a good enough provider for us, having enough room, making sure the air-conditioning is working and the windows are sealed. I tell him I don't need much, and that he's going to be a great dad. I start crying, wiping my eyes with scratchy Mad Greek napkins. He doesn't touch his food, and his hands are shaking a little bit, which only happens when he's really upset.

My nose starts to bleed, just a trickle. My stomach starts to cramp, and I figure this must be one of those Braxton Hicks contractions I've heard about, mild, irregular "practice" contractions that are usually felt by the second or third trimester. I wipe my bloody nose, wipe my eyes, don't mention the cramps because I've just finished assuring my husband there is nothing to worry about, that we won't break down in the desert, that we'll get the windows fixed, that I know he'll provide us with all we need, that he married a girl who cries and bends but doesn't really break.

The wheat bread is toasted on one side and soft on the other, but I eat both pieces. We hit the road.

"This trip is going to be great from now on. I was just worried about getting you there. Now, I'm psyched," Daniel says cheerfully. Soon, I will make him promise to take me to any hospital except the one twenty minutes or so from the Strip. My mom lives in Vegas, so I'm familiar with the place. I have no idea if what is happening to me is serious; all I know is that I don't want to end up at the peach-colored hospital on the outskirts of town, because you go there to die, or at least my stepfather did. When he passed (as Hemingway would say, "gradually and then suddenly"), his death certificate described him as white and his cause of death as leukemia.

Only he was black. And died of congenital heart failure.

Probably an honest mistake, but it doesn't point to great attention to detail. That hospital reminds me of sloppiness and slipping away, and while I have a long history of being lukewarm on my own existence, the pull to keep this baby safe is mooring me to this world like nothing else has.

The cramps abate until right when we exit the I-5 in Vegas. Only now, they are about ten times worse than extreme menstrual cramps, and we are stuck in Friday afternoon congestion. I have to take off my seat belt. I check the clock, and it's been twenty minutes or more of this one cramp. I quietly Google "Braxton Hicks" on my iPhone so as not to panic my husband, and from what I can tell, those are supposed to feel like a mild tightening, but not painful. Another half an hour goes by, which is when I decide to tell my husband, just in case I'm actually having preterm labor.

I'm doubling over now. I'm pretty sure I won't be able to walk through the lobby of the hotel without some help, but I can't spook the Mister because this whole stupid Vegas thing was all my idea and it was obviously completely idiotic.

Somehow, we make it to our room at the Palms. I will myself to walk upright but find myself stopping to lean against slot machines every few yards. We call our doctor, who says I'm probably dehydrated. Drink water and rest, she says, and if things don't improve in two hours, call back.

My husband pours me a bath and I drink all four bottles of Smart Water he bought in the lobby. I soak and listen to CNN and read *USA Today*. In two hours, I'm fine. I glance out the window and look down at the Palms pool, where it's "Ditch Friday," a packed bash the locals call "sweaty ball soup" because of the preponderance of male attendees. Part of me feels like I'm watching children trick-or-treat from behind a curtain, nursing a case of mono, but most of me feels I'm exactly where I should be, cool and safe, away from the blaring Kanye and the pool-friendly canisters of Miller. I was never a party girl before, and you can't go back to a place you've never been, nor should you ever want to dunk yourself into sweaty ball soup.

Often, I wonder what's on the other side of this pregnancy, whether being a parent will be a blissful shuffling of priorities or just something else that's supposed to come naturally to me but doesn't. I can't possibly know how I'll feel once I cross over, but that doesn't stop me from trying to figure it out. One thing that's becoming as clear as the acrylic heels on a showgirl's shoes, the old ways of feeling okay about myself were wearing me out. I'm done grubbing for gold stars to justify being alive, and I wonder if caring for another human being and loving him as well as I can will be gold star enough.

Sitting naked at the desk in the hotel room, cramp-free, my husband rubbing my shoulders, I think I'm almost ready to qualify as a mom, because I've never felt so protective. As long as Buster is okay, I don't care about being a has-been (that barely was), or having kind of a double chin now, or wearing outfits Kate Gosselin would suggest are too "middle America," or gaining forty-five pounds. I don't care that I'm not at the party pool; I don't dance, I've always hated crowds and I burn in the sun. I don't want to be down there, or back home, or in my old body, or anywhere else. My husband demands I drink another bottle of water, and I imagine him with Buster in a Baby-Björn, holding my hand, and I don't know how I ever got out of the desert intact.

I only know that as sure as I can take a wrong turn, I can right myself, usually by just sitting still.

nineteen

Are Breast-Feeding Classes for Boobs?

Here's what you need to know about exclusively breast-fed babies: They can levitate.

That's what I learn during a three-hour breast-feeding class.

They also are immune to disease, are more likely to win Nobel Prizes, recycle, live meaningful lives, understand James Joyce, love fully, donate to NPR pledge drives, stop to help distressed motorists, appreciate Rachmaninoff, have high credit scores, get appointed to important government posts, and have X-ray vision. Oh, and breast-fed babies live forever. The science on that isn't totally in yet, but better safe than sorry.

Moreover, if you breast-feed, the baby weight will melt off of you. You will evade reproductive cancers. The release of the feel-good hormone oxytocin when your baby is "at your breast" will saturate your system with "delicious" feelings of attachment and contentment such as you have never experienced before. Mothers who miss out on this mommy morphine are likely to leave their babies in the middle of the road to be pecked at by turkey vultures.

Okay, that's not totally true. Some mothers who skip this crucial biological bonding experience will simply leave their child in a basket at a fire station with $5 and half a pack of Benson & Hedges Menthol Ultra Lights in a box.

Breast-fed babies will have fewer ear infections, allergies, stomach ailments and a much lower chance of obesity. They will have higher IQ scores. So say the adherents. So says the teacher of this class, a tall, fit, broad-shouldered woman in her fifties who looks like she played high school volleyball.

A room full of us pregnant ladies, shifting around in uncomfortable plastic chairs and gnawing on free cookies with our husbands, are also given a stern warning: Never ever let the baby out of your sight at the hospital once it is born.

Some sleepy, overworked, well-meaning but ultimately venal nurse is going to hear it cry and give it . . . well, what might as well be a cocktail of lead paint, asbestos juice and Southern Comfort: *formula*. That's right, your precious baby's ability to be exclusively fed at your breast, the way god and Mother Nature intended, will be forever compromised if you don't step up with some major vagina power and tell the nurses they are *not* taking your baby out of your sight for one single second at the hospital. Once that baby gets away from you and into the hospital nursery, it's a free-for-all and you can kiss your dreams of attending your child's inauguration good-bye. Once it gets a taste of that plastic nipple and guzzles away at that easy-access bottle, forget that child loving you, crafting you handmade cards or even sitting in your lap.

We also learn some of the more subtle differences between bottle- and breast-fed babies. Like, babies who are bottle-fed stink. They smell foul. As for breast-fed tykes, their shit literally doesn't stink, though it may be an alarming shade of black before it goes mustard yellow and seedy.

That's what I learn in my breast-feeding class.

On the other hand, outside of the beige and pastel pink confines of this breast-feeding store, which is tucked away in an urban strip mall in Hollywood, out in the real mom world, some of my girlfriends just didn't take to breast-feeding, and their kids seem fine. From my unscientific sampling of moms I know who chose to bottle-feed, I see no asthma, no allergies and no bonding problems with the babies. The moms lost the baby weight just fine. I'm not sure if the kids are a ticking time bomb or the moms are just enjoying a few years until the uterine cancer kicks in, but it seems unlikely. I also know mothers who were literally sick with grief when they couldn't breast-feed because their babies had a "weak suck" or they just didn't produce enough of the magical elixir to keep the little ones alive. I'm not sure why these women, who did their best, read every book and took every class, and dragged their newborns to appointments with lactation specialists, should be made to feel selfish and negligent because breast-feeding didn't work out for them.

From where I sit—on my now numb ass—it seems like support groups for breast-feeding women are redundant. This whole culture, at least out here in Los Angeles, supports breast-feeding women. The gals who really need a safe place to compare notes and not have to hide from formula-sniffing dogs and do-gooding busybodies are the formula-feeding moms. There is so much pressure for women to succeed at the boob-feeding that if they fail they feel like they have to hide out so some idiot doesn't spy a packet of powdered Enfamil in their diaper bag and chime in with the now standard "breast is best." I buy that breast is best, but it isn't always possible or practical, and I kind of just think we should stay the hell out of each other's bras.

It's difficult to find an expert or parent who doesn't have a horse in the breast-feeding versus formula race, which makes it hard for us pregnant girls to truly understand our options and their repercussions. To be fair, hard data is difficult to come by, because there are so many variables that go into a child's intelligence, or propensity toward allergies, or ability to bond.

Obviously, an over-Googling, fear-based creature like me is attracted to the idea of inoculating my child against all ills with my magical breasts, but there is also the matter of working to consider. At some point, me and the rest of the employed, semi-employed and hoping or needing to be employed moms in this class won't be able to be around our babies every two to three hours, and though we can pump (they sell all manner of pumps at this store and others), that seems like having a second full-time job. All of this may be—probably is—worth it for the miraculous antibodies breast milk reportedly provides, but it's still a major time "suck" if it works, and a major mouthful of guilt if it doesn't.

Our statuesque teacher, a certified lactation consultant and part owner of the store hosting the class, impresses me with her vast knowledge of boobies and extreme comfort in discussing latching and leaking. She even has a pink velveteen dummy breast, on which she demonstrates various breast-feeding holds. However, when she tells us about her own kids and mentions how healthy the now grown offspring are, she adds that one of them has a little bit of asthma, only when he runs. Wait a second; you mean this panacea doesn't work for someone who was breast-fed for two years?

"The doctors told us it would have been way, way worse if I hadn't breast-fed," she explains.

Really?

Now that is some backward, biased data analysis if I've ever heard it. Look, the kid has respiratory problems and his mom is a lactation lady who did nothing but breast-feed him the "right" way for two years straight. That means one-third of her three children has asthma. How can this fact fit into the hypothesis that breast milk effectively staves off breathing problems? Would it really have been worse without the breast milk? No one can know that for sure, and while I like this woman, and her good posture and better diction, she does seem to be using a logic shoehorn to make sense of her own experience.

Along with the demonstration and lecture, we are also shown a grainy VHS movie, the production values of which can only be compared to an early snuff film, featuring a freckled, naked mother just after giving birth.

Her baby, possibly of German descent but it's hard to tell because there is no dialogue, is placed on her chest and allowed to root around until she finds the nipple. This process takes about half an hour, after which the girl finds the boob and suckles away. I must admit that it's beautiful to see, and who wouldn't want such a natural, easy first nursing experience, a newborn all calm and snuggly on her mother's chest? The lactation lady warns us of the dangers of getting the wrong kind of latch, which would be painful and perhaps impede the child's ability to get enough milk. The imperfect latch could lead to nipple scabbing—for which the store sells plenty of remedies, of course—and we should be careful to gently open the baby's jaw downward and mush the nipple out with our hands so the kid gets kind of a flesh sandwich, with a nice full mouth of both nipple and areola. I start to fade with mental overload and whisper to my husband, "Are you getting this?"

"Yes. Sandwich latch. Got it," he answers, looking down at his watch. The room is stuffy. I notice a couple of the other husbands nodding out, but this isn't latch lady's first day at the sleepy husband rodeo.

"You in the front row, I know you're tired, but stay with me. How often do we nurse a new baby?" she asks a man with disheveled black hair and maroon corduroy pants.

Waking from his accidental slumber, he looks alarmed. His wife whispers something in his ear. "On demand," he mumbles, unsure.

"That's right," she announces, turning her voice up a couple of notches. "When do we nurse a baby? When the baby is hungry. The baby will let you know."

When it's Q & A time, I sheepishly inquire as to how long one should nurse a baby for maximum benefit (subtext, *What's the least amount of time I can nurse a baby before I return to my life without everyone judging me?*). Subtext is not something lactation lady misses. She runs her fingers through her expertly highlighted blond hair and sighs dramatically, clearly unhappy with my tone.

"I don't know your baby yet. All babies are different. The American Academy of Pediatrics recommends breast-feeding for six months exclusively and for the first year with solid foods, but you do what you can." I can't be sure, but from the way she stops looking in my direction for the rest of the class, I think she has dismissed me as someone not seriously dedicated to breast-feeding and already eyeing the finish line before I've even begun. What I'm really eyeing is the El Pollo Loco next door, hoping it will still be open when this shindig ends so I can get a burrito bowl for the road.

I understand the almost religious fervor of these hard-core breast-feeding advocates. If I had to take a side, it would be theirs.

There was a time when women were essentially forced to bottle-feed by doctors and hospitals and prevented from caring for their babies in a way that seems both best for the baby (even if only marginally) and righteous. Breast-feeding was once seen as low-class, while mothers of means chose the bottle and were proud to do so, because they could afford it and because the prevailing wisdom was that formula was more "hygienic."

There was a time when the hospital knocked moms out, yanked your baby away from you after birth and generally ignored what we now understand to be the importance of skin-to-skin contact, bonding, nursing right after birth, and so on. Betty Draper and her real-life counterparts got screwed, for sure. At this point, however, it seems the pendulum may have swung too far in the other direction, so that women for whom breast-feeding just doesn't make sense or feel right, or for whom it's physically impossible, are vilified as selfish, lazy, impatient baby haters. Intolerance stinks worse than a formula-fed baby's poop. It stinks on both sides of the intolerance diaper.

Look, I'm going to give breast-feeding a try, and I hope it works. But if it doesn't happen, or if maybe I'm not the nurse-for-two-years kind of girl, I hope the milk of human kindness is also available in formula.

twenty

Sitting Stretch Mark *Shiva*

I have a stretch mark.

This is not a big deal. Or rather, I wish I were a person for whom this was not a big deal, but after spending two hours online in the middle of the night looking at pictures of stretch marks, I realize I do not subscribe to the Warrior Woman thing about "my trophy" and "all worth it" and "this was my baby's home for nine months." Fuck that.

Did I mention I just have the one? Still, it's red and loud like a blinking, broken arrow, an arrow pointing right to the place where my vanity lives, a tenant I expected to be evicted and replaced by groovy, maternal "Don't care how I look because I'm so in love with motherhood" Lady. Whether depth and vanity can share a home without finishing off each other's peanut butter or bogarting the laundry detergent, I have no idea.

I just know I took a long look at the mark in the mirror in the middle of the night and had a racking, choking cry.

The cute part of pregnancy is over. It came to a conclusive and crashing end when I bought a five-pack of extra-large underpants. It was over when I had to go to the mall jewelry store and have my wedding rings cut off my finger because my hands are so swollen that even dipping them in a mixture of dishwashing soap and Astroglide couldn't coax the rings over my knuckles. Yeah, this stopped being divine when I hit up the discount shoe store for some emergency size tens to wear on *The Dr. Phil Show* (exploiting my baby in daytime) to do a segment about baby names. Size *tens*. I was shooting a "man-on-the-street" piece asking passersby what to name my baby, looking like a pregnant Minnie Mouse in an orange dress and giant flat shoes. When I see the segment on TV, I look like a traffic cone with jowls.

My boobs are leaking a little, I haven't seen my vagina in weeks and getting around the back to wipe my own ass has become a geometry problem of sorts. I would need a protractor and a better grasp of math to explain it, but trust me, the angles don't add up to wiping with ease. There's only so fast I can dash out of a room to create some distance between myself and the gas that I can no longer control, but I try, because I don't have or want the kind of relationship that involves "Dutch ovens" or any other form of gas humor. As far as I'm concerned, there should be no shared experience of gas in our marriage. I don't even want him to read this chapter later. So, let's just say outrunning my own gas has replaced the treadmill as my new form of cardio.

My doctor says most women get a rush of stretch marks in the last weeks before childbirth, and I think I see several more appearing on the left side of my stomach, crouching, lying in wait to ambush my collagen and my confidence. My twice-daily stretch mark prevention protocol is beginning to involve more and more steps. There's the natural oil from the health food store, sealed in with the expensive

Crème de la Mer body cream my pregnant friend Cassandra recommended, finished off with a third layer of stretch mark cream that was suggested online and is so goopy you have to warm it up by rubbing your palms together before you can even try spreading it across your belly. I smell like a combination of high-priced call girl and Whole Foods cashier. Most of my clothes now feature both sweat and oil stains, like a good mechanic's.

My goddamn dermis, like everything else in my body, is out of my hands, no matter how much goop is in my hands.

If you search long enough, you can find anything online, like sites that encourage moms to post pictures of their bellies, with or without stretch marks, and tell their stories. It is very disturbing, these women who look like they've been clawed across the abdomen by a giant, angry bear and their own genetics. I want to find them valiant but just see my own mother, practically disfigured by groups of chunky, textured, silvery marks. It never seemed to bother her much, which made it bother me more, and maybe the entire process of looking in the mirror and seeing my mother triggers a deep Freudian crisis. How am I supposed to keep repressing the idea that I'll become her emotionally when I'm slowly becoming her physically, staring at the empirical evidence etched across my abdomen? If there is no meaningful link between how she took to motherhood and how I will, why am I wearing it?

I also find photos of women who escaped pregnancy unscathed, not a mark on their bellies. Well, goooooood for you, says my mind in the quiet calm of the night, goooood for you.

Of course, I still worry about big things, too.

I worry all the time about the baby being born deaf or blind or not making it at all. I worry that I have tempted fate with my Diaper

Champ and my hand-me-down crib and my drawers full of onesies, as if to say to the universe that I take it for granted I will get a real, live baby.

Old-fashioned superstition has been preventing me from having a baby shower, but at the last minute, I cave. I need things, and one of those things may just be the sense that I can do normal mom activities, like have a shower. My girlfriend Lynette throws it for me, and it's coed, just friends meeting for drinks, really. The only "tell" that it's a baby shower at all is a tower of blue frosted cupcakes decorated with rattles and stuffed bears. I have half a glass of wine and come away with things moms tell me I'll need: a tiny blue plastic tub, a play mat, diaper bags and the like.

A few times a day, I'm scared to have those things, and I still hold out on buying diapers, as if it's some sort of unilateral negotiation with the Big Guy not to screw me over. See, I don't really take it for granted that I will have a healthy baby, or I would have a closet full of Pampers. I know it's twisted, but no one can accuse me of only worrying about superficial things like stretch marks. As a Jew, I have enough room in my *kishkes* for all levels of anxiety. The shelves are stocked with sizes from XS to XXL. I'm ready for this to be over, not just so I can stem the rising tide of worries and wounds, but so I can escape the restlessness.

I just want this kid out so I can sleep on my back without suffocating, roll over in bed without sounding like Fred Sanford, not be congested anymore, smoke a couple cigarettes on a Friday night or when I'm writing and need to feel like Norman Mailer. I want to drink a freezing cold martini, fit into my old shoes, schedule toxic beauty treatments. Most of all, I want to be done wondering if Buster is all right, if he'll survive his passage out of my body, if I did a good enough job carrying him for all these months, if he got all his omega fatty acids and protein and folic acid and fat and brain stimulation. Like probably everyone who is pregnant for the first time and close to the end, I just want to hold my baby.

Maybe, as I spit blood from my swollen gums every time I brush my teeth (pregnancy gingivitis) and stare at my pudgy, terrified face in the mirror and wake in the night to stare at my belly by the dim light of a floor lamp, it's easier to focus on one single stretch mark. There's only so far it can rip you apart.

This facile psychological interpretation not only buys me a one-way ticket to obvious-ville, it makes me look so much better than a woman who hyperventilates over a stretch mark.

Or maybe a stretch mark breakdown is simply that. The fact is, these suckers are truly irreversible. Maybe I just need a second to let it register.

They can send a man to the moon, transplant a human face, smash an atom with a linear accelerator, air-condition a condo in Phoenix, make sure you always know exactly where you are in space with a $200 GPS the size of a wallet. Yet they can't really do much about the scars of motherhood.

I don't want this one stretch mark. I don't want more. I don't want to spend the rest of my life self-consciously tugging down T-shirts so there's no flesh-exposing gap between the bottom of my shirt and the waist of my jeans. I don't want to wear matronly swimsuits. Just thinking this makes me feel like a baby, and the fact is, I can't be a baby anymore because I'm going to have to care for one. This is the rub that comes with no lotion: I have to wear my big-girl pants now, and they can't be low-rise.

Every transition involves a loss; even if you are blessed enough to find yourself pregnant and on the eve of motherhood and the luckiest darn thirty-nine-year-old alive, there is still something left behind, and even if that something is just a silly image of yourself looking halfway decent in a bikini, one thing is giving way to another and it can't hurt to stop and wave good-bye.

In my own way, I have to sit *shiva*, grieve a bit for what was and allow myself to be fully and fairly alarmed and inspired by what's coming.

That or just get some self-tanner.

People I Want to Punch: People Who Won't Tell Me What to Do

I t's a recurring theme, me wanting answers from the outside, resisting a dip in Lake Teresa, where I can never seem to tell if it's too cold or too hot or just plain polluted. When people tell me that only *I* know what's right for me, I want to punch them until they tell me what *they* think is right for me.

Now I've got to figure out where to live, a decision I have been putting off ever since I found out I was pregnant.

Stay put, or move? As you can imagine, no matter how many people I poll about my housing options, I get the same infuriating response: "Depends." Next time someone says that word, they better be referring to the brand of adult diapers they are going to wear after I administer a beating so brutal they'll think twice before saying the "right" thing instead of attempting to run my life for me. Man, I really do want to punch people who I suspect know what I should do but refuse to tell me.

So, what do you think I should do?

When I was single, I bought a cheap, drafty Craftsman-style house in the Koreatown section of Los Angeles, a ninety-seven-year-old "fixer-upper" with three bedrooms and one bathroom. The plumbing was jacked up, the roof was on its last tarry legs, the exterior paint was peeling and chipping like a bad manicure, but it was mine, transforming me from renter to owner. In the winter, it was so cold I pulled a space heater right up to my bed, slept in my bathrobe and Uggs with two cats and still woke up with purple hands and frozen feet. In the summer, I slept with three fans and a mobile air-conditioning unit that eventually imploded.

Over time, I made improvements, stripping layers of lime green paint from the wooden beams and staining them a deep brown, ripping out the decayed kitchen linoleum and laying in cork floors, replacing the drooping rosewood slat ceilings with drywall.

Still, there wasn't much I could do about the neighborhood, which in some ways was a step down from my old haunt in East Hollywood, the Village of the Damned.

My little section of K-town features several halfway houses and a massive single-room-occupancy building for formerly homeless ex-cons trying to reenter society. There are always mattresses on the sidewalk and guys going through trash for bottles and cans to add to their overfilled shopping carts. Basically, it's District 9. To give you a sense of how dodgy it is, not one restaurant will even deliver food to my block.

I was no stranger to ghettos, but the place was big and scary for a single girl, so when I could afford it, I bought a small condo in Los Feliz, a much nicer neighborhood, and rented out the old place in Koreatown. The new digs dazzled me with things I had never had before in my life: a dishwasher, central heat and air, windows without bars.

When I got married, Daniel moved in with me, and though it was cramped, we pimped it out with a flat-screen television mounted on the bedroom wall, and now we never stop uttering the same annoying phrase: "We can park on a Friday and not get back in our cars until Monday morning. This neighborhood has everything."

Still, with the two of us barely fitting in the space, we wonder where we would put the baby. The second bedroom, which we had turned into an office, shares a wall with the master bedroom. Will nine hundred square feet be enough for the three of us? Can we even fit a crib into that office without getting rid of the desk? How are we supposed to know what life will be like with a baby? We know absolutely nothing about babies, nurseries, how much room baby gear takes up, how loud they cry, or how much they alienate crotchety neighbors.

Of course, I run this dilemma by everyone I know: Stay in our nice condo and be on top of each other, or move back into the 'hood, install a climate control system, and have enough space for a nursery (and plenty of empty, abandoned lots nearby where the phrase "Megan's Law" gets the locals scurrying for cover)?

"It's up to you," everyone answers, along with some variation on, "You just have to decide if you prefer living where you can safely walk around or if you want the extra room."

With every answer Socratically pointing the question right back at me, I want to thrust my fist toward the person's jaw and just yell, "Tell me what to do or I'll smash your face in! Just tell me!"

This goes on for months. I ask parents of small children, I ask crystal balls, I ask my therapist and relatives, but as my due date gets closer, all I do is walk around the quaint streets of Los Feliz and go over and over the intricacies of the decision with Daniel, weighing everything from mortgage costs to moving costs. We get estimates on heat and air, which are all over the place and can make your head explode like my old a/c unit.

Finally, we figure it out. And that's how I end up moving back to the old place, almost nine months pregnant, on a hundred-degree day.

I'm working at this point, so Daniel and the movers handle everything until I get there in the late afternoon. He begs me to stay away, check into a hotel or something, but as anyone who has moved knows, no matter how much help you get, there are still things that only you can do.

The process of moving, of handling every single thing you own and deciding whether it's relevant to your current lifestyle while reminiscing about how you acquired it, not only makes you sweat your balls off (I have balls now; they are just inside me and belong to Buster), it also causes a kind of existential crisis. Who am I? you ask yourself with every object packed or discarded. Am I a person who needs a collection of ceramic cowgirls and more than one pepper grinder? Do I hold on to yellowing clips of stories I wrote for newspapers ten years ago, or let them go? How many pairs of tall brown boots will serve the person I'm going to be from here on out? Do I keep the novelty key chain with a picture of my ex-boyfriend and me, or should I just go ahead and store the memory in my brain and not the key chain in an old cigar box?

We have taken to watching a cable show about hoarders, which leads to our favorite new catchphrase, "That's something a hoarder would do." When I pack a half-empty package of paper plates, my husband points out, "That's something a hoarder would do." When he eyeballs a threadbare Phillies bath towel before folding it and sticking it in a box, I stop him before it lands with a pointed, "That's something a hoarder would do."

As I sit on a pile of cardboard boxes that must all be unpacked, perspiring through my bright yellow sleeveless maternity dress, I announce that this is the worst day of my life and start crying.

The movers go about their business, only slightly fazed by the giant pregnant lady perched on a box, moaning. My husband reassures me this will just be one bad day, after which we'll be grateful for the extra room. He has hired a guy to install central heat and air, so there is sawing and hammering, dust particles flying through the soon-to-be-cooled air.

We never should have waited until the last second. I know this, and I blame myself. Well, I blame myself and punch myself emotionally, but I also idiotically blame all those who didn't tell me to move sooner. If I ask your advice and you have a hunch about what I should do, just hit me with it. If not, I'll want to hit you.

twenty-one

Frank Swoops in to Save My Vagina

On the upper-right-hand corner of the screen during one of my final pre-birth ultrasounds, I see the name Frank Breech.

"Who the fuck is that?" I ask myself. I'm aware that pregnancy can cause cognitive shrinkage, or so-called baby brain, but I swear, *I don't even know him.* That is neither my baby's name nor my husband's name. Is that my doctor? I could have sworn my ob-gyn was an Asian lady named Ann, not some dude named Frank.

More on my confusion about Frank Breech later, because while I don't know him, he has a big say on the future outcome of both my vagina and taint.

First I should remind you that every single ultrasound I've had, I'm so sure the baby's heart has stopped that I hold my breath until I see the organ squeezing and pumping. I mainly think about how much it would suck to be either the doctor or the ultrasound tech, to have to break it to unfortunate couples that instead of a little gestating bundle of joy they have a nonviable fetus.

A dead baby.

It was one thing to worry about *dead baby* before that CVS test, when it was just another one of my loony phobias, but since then I'm a maniac. When the spider actually bites you, your arachnophobia doesn't exactly clear up. Sure, it wasn't my dead baby, but it was right there in the next room.

Every single time they fire up that sonogram machine, I just think about the ultrasound technician, and how she puts on those Crocs and lavender scrubs and intersects with the best and worst days in people's lives. I wonder if she gets sick of people making the same idiotic jokes about their male fetus and his giant penis (because I notice all boy parents joke about the huge phallus they think they see). And I wonder if she has some sort of script she uses for the dead baby days. Most of all, I wonder if on those dead baby days she stops by Chili's on the way home for some fajitas to go, grabs a bottle of $10 pinot from the corner liquor store and drains her DVR of old episodes of *Oprah* while bingeing on flour tortillas, because that's what I would do, perhaps capping off the night with half an Ambien.

I'm splayed out with that clear gel smeared on my stomach repeating my usual silent prayer, "No dead baby. No dead baby. No dead baby. No dead baby. No dead baby." For a second, just reading her face, I'm convinced this poor woman is going to have to slowly walk her Crocs out the door after saying something innocuous, but obviously doomsday, like "I'll be right back" before getting the doctor to break it to me about the *dead baby*.

So you can see why I'm distracted when trying to process this Frank Breech thing. As soon as I stop envisioning the tech scraping the remains of her Chili's dinner into the trash and tucking in for the night with her cat, Mr. Whiskers, I realize I've heard the word "breech" before. I remember from one of my pregnancy books that breech is bad, something about the baby being in the wrong position.

The doctor comes in and explains that a frank breech baby is one whose rump is aimed toward the birth canal, the legs sticking up in front of the body with the hips flexed and feet near his ears. The boy is supposed to be head-down.

This explains all the hiccups I have been feeling up near my ribs, because the baby's head is right up there, where it shouldn't be.

The doctor tells me she can try to turn him, a process called external cephalic version, during which she manually rotates the baby—a process that's nearly always attempted in a hospital in case an emergency C-section is required because of fetal distress. It carries a small risk of cord entanglement or damage to the placenta, it can be quite painful, and when I ask her how often it works, she tucks her hair behind her ear, bites her lower lip and answers, "About half the time."

This is the first appointment I've gone to without my husband and I wish he were here, because what my doctor has called a "one-page" pregnancy—meaning there have been so few complications my whole chart doesn't exceed one page—is about to be continued on page two. I can tell it's a big deal, because the doc is now settling in on a vinyl stool near the window and she has that "we're going to be here for a while" look. She cracks open a Diet Coke.

The umbilical cord could be wrapped around his neck, she says, or there could be some other reason my baby is all ass-backward.

I feel protective about my boy, Frank, and I don't understand much about the situation but I know for certain I don't want to start shoving him around.

She calls in the receptionist. We schedule a C-section. Just like that. It's on the books.

If the key to happiness is wanting what you have instead of having what you want, I need a locksmith. While I was dreading the torn taint, the mad dash to the hospital, the unimaginable pain of labor and vaginal childbirth, now I feel horribly cheated out of all those things. Before I had my very own C-section on the docket, scheduled like a routine dental exam, the whole idea of a Cesarean section was actually pretty appealing, taking something wildly unpredictable like childbirth and making it controlled and contained. Now, I'm sure that I'm getting the shaft; that this is the worst c-word of all. As I maneuver my car out of the parking lot of the doctor's office and call my husband to tell him about our son, Frank, my voice starts to crack.

Saying I cry a lot is like saying Lindsay Lohan has been exposed to a lot of unfiltered UVB rays; it's patently obvious, so it's difficult to discuss my emotional lows and lows without being redundant. Suffice to say, I bawled through my explanation and vowed to look into some of the alternate, noninvasive methods of turning him mentioned by the doctor: acupuncture, yoga, bags of cold peas and music.

The rest of the day I spend stewing in jealousy for every woman who has given birth the way nature intended. I want my water break-ing at Pilates or in the middle of the night. I want to rush out the door with my prepacked hospital bag and the Mister nervously speeding along his rehearsed route. I want my own gory story, hours spent push-ing, epidural, no epidural, eating ice chips, cursing, rolling on one of those giant plastic workout balls with my doula gently coaching me to breathe. I want reports on how I'm dilating and effacing so I can Tweet the whole event between contractions, exploiting my baby as he enters the world. I want to walk around and around the block to help the contractions along, have sex to bring on labor, eat this special salad they serve at a restaurant in the Valley that's supposed to make your water break. That moment when the painful pushing is over, and the little guy squirms out into his father's arms, I won't have that mo-ment. If one could give birth to self-pity, however, I would be deliver-ing a litter at this point.

Pooooooooor me. Just a small percentage of women have breech babies, and I am one of them.

Even though my gut tells me this is it, frankly, there is still time for the baby to turn, so I try to encourage him to do so.

Moxibustion is a Chinese technique that consists of burning sticks made from the herb moxa on or near an acupuncture point on the little toe of each foot. This is supposed to stimulate the production of maternal hormones, which make the uterus contract, which can make the baby turn. People love acupuncture, and I love it in theory, but every time I've tried it there's a whole lot of expensive sitting around with needles in you and frustration you have to choke down like the bogus fistfuls of Chinese herbs they give you. Seriously, I don't want to go all Western medicine on you, but if a lady with a medical degree isn't sure she can physically turn my baby with her well-trained hands, burning some herbs near my toes half a dozen times just feels like something that's likely to cause more disappointment than baby flipping.

There are yoga positions recommended for turning breech babies—getting on all fours, getting in a modified plank. I try all that stuff, but mostly just find it brings on acid reflux. Then there's the theory you can coerce the baby out by putting frozen peas up top so he'll want to escape the chilly climes and inch downward. That pea enterprise is as cold, long and sad as *Dr. Zhivago*. I even combine the two, getting on all fours with a bag of frozen peas strapped to my ribs. While this makes a spectacular "How would I explain this to an alien?" moment, it doesn't seem to be a baby turner.

Some experts say another way to cajole the baby into a head-down position so he can safely dive out vaginally is to place headphones toward the mom's pubic bone and play music for ten minutes, six to eight times a day. Could the right song list played near my girl parts save me a major surgery and an unsightly scar? If I lure him down south through the majesty of song, will I get the chaotic, exciting, vaginal birth I suddenly feel I must have?

This begs the obvious question, what songs? I ask for suggestions from my blog readers and Twitter followers and get some excellent selections.

"Into the Great Wide Open" **by Tom Petty**

"Down in the Hole" **by the Rolling Stones**

"Jump Around" **by House of Pain**

"Follow You Down" **by the Gin Blossoms**

"Hold On, I'm Coming" **by Sam and Dave**

"Head On" **by the Pixies**

"Heading Out to the Highway" **by Judas Priest**

"Relax" **by Frankie Goes to Hollywood**

"Upside Down" **by Diana Ross**

"We Gotta Get Out of this Place" **by the Animals**

"Turn! Turn! Turn!" **by the Byrds**

My V has a DJ, but still, that baby does not spin.

The doctor tells me that right before they slice you open and remove the baby, they do one last ultrasound to check his position. Every once in a while, you get a last-minute reprieve; the kid has turned and they send you home to wait for labor or induce you right there on the spot. Now, all there is to do is wait. Wait and blast House of Pain and hope that I won't be living in one.

People I Want to Punch: Barkley

I n the middle of the night, I feel something wet next to me in bed.

If my water breaks before my scheduled C-section, it could be trouble. To prevent infection you're supposed to get the kid out within a short amount of time after the amniotic sac ruptures. With my baby breech, we would need to rush into an operating room to pry him loose stat. Now, I'm in a panic trying to figure out the genesis of this mystery moisture.

I quickly rule out any kind of standard pregnancy discharge, because the liquid is neither viscous nor colored in any way. If I had wet myself, and trust me, I was a hard-core bed wetter until my early twenties, so I'm familiar with the sensation, there would be the warm stinging of urine on my inner thighs and, of course, the stench.

I wake Daniel.

"Dude, I think my water broke. Look," I whisper, showing him the wet spot on the white sheet, near my stomach, about the size of a place mat.

He smells it. It's not pee, he agrees. We scramble around for *What to Expect When You're Expecting*, head toward the trusty index and look up "water breaking." Heidi says amniotic fluid should smell like bleach. We sniff the spot again with this in mind. Daniel rouses from bed in his T-shirt and plaid flannel pajama pants and rips the sheet from the bed so he can investigate it further.

The color is clear, as amniotic fluid often is, but we don't really smell the bleachlike odor that the alkaline liquid is supposed to have.

"Give me your panties," demands my husband. I wince.

"No. You are *not* smelling my panties. Please don't make me let you smell my panties. What if there's something gross going on?" I plead, standing there in my black maternity nightgown with crazy hair looking like a combination troll doll–bowling ball. I don't even like him touching my dirty laundry and I generally feel strongly about trying to maintain some of my feminine mystique.

"This is a medical situation," he says sternly. "Give me the panties."

"Fine. I'll smell my own panties. You stay away," I say, slipping them off and turning my back to him as I sniff. Nothing. My extra-large flesh-colored cotton underpants are dry with no notable scent.

So how does a patch of odorless, colorless liquid

end up on the sheet right under me in the middle of the night when I'm a full-term pregnant lady? This must be significant. It must be something. If it walks like a duck, quacks like a duck, it's a . . . cat? Could Barkley, my no-good nuisance of a tabby, have been responsible? Daniel notices an empty plastic tumbler that has rolled under the bed. It doesn't take Nancy Drew to figure out that Barkley knocked over the cup of water that had been on the nightstand. With feline grace, she managed to dump all the contents right on the bed and let the cup gently roll over the side without waking either of us up.

You know how on the morning news they regularly feature animals from a local shelter and encourage viewers to adopt them? I was doing that very segment one morning on *Good Day New York*, holding a three-week-old orphaned kitten and asking viewers to visit the shelter in Queens and give her a good home. When we threw to commercial, the cat was still on my shoulder, nervously digging her claws into my blazer, and I thought, "Oh, shit. I guess she's mine now." I took her home, got her a tiny bottle because she was too young to eat solid foods, and raised her up to be an obese and troublesome ingrate who has now aggravated me on both coasts. The first week I had her, she tried to jump into a hot bath twice, stuck her whiskers into a lit candle and ate so much milk she toppled over. Okay, that one was my fault for overfeeding her, but her troublemaking ways earned her a name inspired by one of my favorite basketball players, Charles Barkley. The Round Mound from the Pound has ripped my arm to shreds when she didn't care for being placed in her cardboard carrier, she has hissed at delivery people just trying to pet her head, she has refused all but one brand of food, and she once barely missed my eye while gouging my cheek when I tried to brush out her matted fur.

Now, she's really done it.

I dole out my usual threat about taking her back to the pound to be put down. "One more stunt like this and you're off to Meowschwitz, lady." I cool down a bit. "All right, Barkley, any more shenanigans from you and I'm taking you to a nice no-kill shelter in the suburbs."

She's woken us up, made me smell my own panties, made us rush around in the wee hours thinking the baby was coming and all because she thinks it's delightful to swat objects from the table and watch them fall. I should have named her Newton, because she seems to discover gravity every day.

I can't get back to sleep now, and it's the usual fidgeting around, trying to shove my pillows and my body into a comfortable position. Instead of restorative sleep, I kind of fantasize about getting revenge on Barkley. Not punching her, of course, because for one thing that's cruel and for another I would never get in the ring with that beast because she's fourteen pounds of fury, but I wouldn't mind locking her out for the night and letting her experience the biting cold chill of Los Angeles in September, a frigid sixty-five degrees.

To keep her from coming back into our bedroom,

we wedge one of my husband's flip-flops under the door, which she has figured out how to open.

We're not worried she'll attack the baby, as she seems to be very scared of children and generally avoids them. But if Barkley is any indication of the type of parent I will become, look out, juvenile hall, because my disciplinary style, at least when it comes to bad cats, is a mixture of blind love and empty threats. My water hasn't broken, but my resolve has. After a few minutes, I pry loose the shoe and let Barkley back in, where she takes her usual spot across Daniel's knees.

twenty-two

Seinfeld Curbs My Enthusiasm

With the help of Jerry Seinfeld, I am going to exploit Buster all the way to network prime-time television.

I didn't get *The View* years back because I had no child, but screw that, because I'm going to be part of Seinfeld's triumphant return to TV and all thanks to the fetus. This new show is all hush-hush, but my agent tells me Jerry is creating a new reality program about marriage and that the host, a popular stand-up comedian who regularly opens for Seinfeld, needs a female sidekick.

Sidekicking is my thing, did it for years with Carolla.

As well as being in-studio with a panel of celebrities commenting on an arguing married couple, the female cohost will be sent out to do short comedic "man on the street"–type pieces to bump in and out of commercials. The job will be part correspondent, part second banana, laughing at the host's jokes, throwing in a fact or two, keeping the talk ball in the air. These are all things I've done before.

"You're sure they know I'm pregnant?" I ask my agent, driving over to the meeting. "And you're sure they still want to meet me?" Yes, she tells me for the ninth time, reminding me that their shooting schedule means that by the time they need me, Buster will be three months old. It's perfect, she says. Still, I've got a C-section on the books in a week, I look like I'm in my seventh trimester, they have to know I'm going to be a bit distracted with a new baby and there is no way they are seriously going to consider hiring me when they could just as easily get a hundred other girls who are younger, prettier, funnier and not even remotely pregnant. *Not that there's anything wrong with that.*

As I'm sitting in a conference room chatting it up with the comedian host and the executive producer, both parents, I sense that even though I'm certain they won't hire me, I'm being kind of . . . charming. We're sitting having a nice casual conversation about babies, pregnancy and deliveries and without meaning to I'm being rather amusing. I don't need them to love me, approve of me, hire me or even laugh at anything I say, because I'm so distracted by Buster and his imminent arrival. I forget to be self-conscious and socially awkward. I forget to try too hard, or I just plain lack the energy. I'm patting my stomach, which is now getting Braxton Hicks contractions almost all the time, while carrying on the most relaxed conversation a girl could have while interviewing for a potentially life-changing job. Not only have I found a new comfort in my own stretched skin, I have the one quality that attracts mates, employers and friends like no other: I don't care.

Wow, I've stumbled into a way of exploiting my baby I hadn't even known was possible. I'm not talking about the boon of creating an affinity with other parents, though it is nice to have a ready topic of conversation for the rest of my life. I'm talking about something more internal. At nine months pregnant, for the first time in my life I'm easy like a Sunday morning. Stage fright in its many forms has plagued me my entire career, a smorgasbord of anxiety, embarrassment and self-doubt. I used to leave auditions in tears if I stumbled over a single word. Now, suddenly, I think I have some perspective.

Don't get too excited; I'm not talking about the abnegation of ego, just perspective enough to give me focus and take away anxiety. I'm working on making Buster an almost fully functioning immune system and he's making me the Master of My Own Emotional Domain.

Leaving that meeting, tottering on my high heels and guzzling water, I think, "Jeez. That was so painless. What nice people. What nice people that will never, ever hire me for this particular job because that would be insane." Still, I touch my cramping belly, the outside of which now feels hard, like a thin candy coating, and thank Buster for making the meeting so stress-free.

If I usually have such terrible stage fright, you may be asking yourself why I would choose this line of work. One answer is that I have very few other skills. Besides that, while working in television and radio may be especially nerve-racking, there's no question I'd get anxious giving a presentation on quarterly earnings, teaching first grade, arguing in front of a jury, reconciling a company's accounts, or trying to sell you a house. So what's the diff? At least this way I can occasionally get the applause and public approval my childhood set me up to need and generally avoid sitting in a cubicle.

It's not always so bad, but I've never found a way to totally overcome it. Of course I've gotten lots of advice. Deep breathing. Visualization. The most frequent prescription: "Just be yourself."

A side note on "Just be yourself":

Well-adjusted people who unabashedly like themselves think this is all you need to hear. Just *be yourself* and all will be well. As if we insecure, bumbling, stage-fright-y bundles of tics were simply lacking this one critical piece of information. As if telling a smoker nicotine causes cancer will suddenly make him stump out his cigarette and make it his last. "What? This is bad for me? Thanks so much for letting me know. I'm going to quit now." We Albert Brooks in *Broadcast News* types fully understand people will like us better if we could "just be ourselves," but we can no more tackle that little bit of psychological business than a smoker can quit just because it's a good idea. We know. Stop telling us something we know, because it only reminds us that our own minds and bodies are engaged in a mutiny, preventing us from doing the one simple thing that could change our fates.

We understand the concept. When we're hanging out having a drink with friends, making the table laugh, not concerned with our phrasing or how our arm looks draped over the back of the chair or whether we're using the word "like" too often, we register that if we could just pull this off in high-pressure situations like dates and interviews, if we could just re-create this sense of flow when it really counted, we would be fine. But for whatever reason—childhood pressure to succeed, painful past failures, brain chemistry explosions, overthinking, overcaffeinating, poor expectation management, whatever—we get that first shot of adrenaline and it's "bring on the shakes and odd, inappropriate remarks and dry mouth," because we can no longer "just be ourselves." To a jittery person, everything is an emergency. Our brains can't differentiate between a tsunami and a callback for a dog food commercial. My nervous system isn't at all sure that pogroms aren't coming to my village or a saber-toothed tiger isn't approaching to eat me.

So frankly, "be yourself" is idiotic advice that doesn't take into account that people with performance anxiety are experiencing autonomic nervous system responses beyond our control.

Aside from which, if you aren't so sure you like yourself, or that others do, this little aphorism is even more inane. Why would we want to "be ourselves" if we don't always particularly like ourselves?

And what does it really mean to "be yourself," anyway? If you are anything but the simplest of one-dimensional dingbats, your "self" is a multifaceted concept, malleable, up for grabs. When I think, "Teresa, just be yourself," I honestly have no idea what that means. Sure, there's the happy-go-lucky me that surfaces under the right conditions (and dosages), there's the generous me that helps elderly neighbors fill out tax forms, but there are lots of other versions that are just as "real," and not so great. *Be myself.* The girl who spends twenty minutes pondering whether she should order her frozen yogurt flavors side by side or twisted? That self? Or how about the one who rambles and repeats herself after tuning out during cocktail party conversations? I know, how about the self who gets a headache in her eyeballs when speaking to any authority figure? Wait, do you want me to be the girl from Monday, who listens patiently to her friend's boy problems, or the girl from Thursday, who can't return a call because she's worried she'll have nothing to say. Even if I *could* just "be myself," I would have to land on a version of "myself" I and others find appealing. It's relatability roulette, and the house always wins.

Don't even get me started on "Just have fun with it."

So, I was just being myself and just having fun with it, and the meeting must have gone pretty well, because within a few hours the producers call to say they want me to screen-test for the job. First, they will send a crew to shoot a brief "man on the street" piece in which I will ask tourists and passersby questions about marriage. The day after that, we will do a full run-through of the show in-studio for Jerry. *Seinfeld.*

At this point, I could go into labor at any moment. Technically,

Buster is full term. And now the producers want me to stand outside talking to strangers on camera for about four hours at Universal Studios in the Valley, where it will be hovering around one hundred degrees.

The radio job has ended, the television show has been canceled, my trust fund is that my parents *trust* that I will *fund* them when they get old, so I figure, why not? I'm going to need a job.

Of course, I want to be safe about it. The morning of the screen test, I go to my doctor's office to get the medical go-ahead, but I'm confident she'll sign off (pregnant women around the world do far more strenuous tasks than audition to cohost a television show, and despite all my complaining, there isn't anything especially risky about this pregnancy). I'm confident that after phase two of my screen test, I will go in to have Buster removed right on schedule, just after he has helped snare me a big job, thus ensuring his own financial future and his mom's sense of relevance. Consider Operation Exploit My Baby deployed in a major way.

Before my doctor can give me clearance, she tells me she has to check to see if I'm dilated.

"Guess you've heard all about this," she says, pulling a glove on her hand.

"Huh?" I ask, because I honestly have no idea what she's talking about. Now she's painted herself into a bedside manner corner and has no choice but to finish her thought.

"Oh, lots of women think this test is painful, but some don't mind at all."

The doctor—and I could get fancy describing this but I won't— jams her fingers into my privates in a move so excruciating my eyes water like I've just rubbed wasabi into my corneas. She announces that I'm dilated about one centimeter. Just the sound of this is thrilling, especially in combination with the procedure ending. There is very little chance that natural labor will take hold in the next few days, but at least I get to *dilate* and get to engage in discussions about effacing and centimeters and all the stuff vaginal delivery girls get to do. My doctor consults with her partners, all working moms, and they tell me if I'm not uncomfortable, there is no reason I shouldn't go to my audition that day. Some people stay at this early phase of labor for weeks, so there's no cause for alarm. They tell me to stay hydrated and maybe to bring my husband, just in case. I go right from the doctor's office to the screen test, toting sunscreen, six bottles of water and Daniel.

That's how I end up standing near the entrance of a crowded theme park, holding a mic and asking couples questions like, "Would you mind if he didn't wear his wedding ring?" and "Should married couples always sleep in the same bed?"

Once again, I'm exploiting my baby for an unprecedented sense of peace and ease. What do I care if Jerry Seinfeld thinks I'm funny? I'm dilating. Huge life changes are happening—there is physical proof! So when it comes to worrying if my retorts and comments and follow-up questions are what the producers want, I'm free and laidback. In fact, I continue to "just have fun with it" and pretty much "just be myself."

One of the problems with this particular self, however, is that it features major boundary problems and a total lack of discretion.

I'm standing out there, just about as pregnant as I can be, and these strangers I'm interviewing couldn't be nicer to me, because of the baby, because I'm out working with a giant bump and without an inch of shade. It's a relentless stream of beaming tourists asking me when I'm due and loving me, loving Buster, really. Sometimes, strangers don't enjoy doing these stupid interviews, because they would rather spend their time buying T-shirts or drinking a beer, but when you exploit your baby just by being enormous, they have endless patience. They laugh extra heartily at your little quips, making you seem even more likeable, more approachable, and more perfect to provide that feminine touch Seinfeld needs for his show.

The crew, the tourists, they are eating up the fact that I'm out here hosting while dilated, which I won't shut up about. My husband is off on a nearby bench trying to conduct business from his phone, keeping an eye on me and my water intake, while I'm yapping about my vagina to anyone who will listen.

"When are you due?" asks every mark we rope in for our interviews.

"Right now. I'm actually dilated as we speak. Yeah, technically, I'm in labor, but it's a very early stage of labor, so don't worry, I won't break my water on your shoes."

I'm exploiting my baby for the adoration of these interviewees and cameramen and sound guys. I'm exploiting him to make myself seem game and sturdy and fun yet vulnerable and maternal. I'm exploiting him for his ability to make me stop caring whether I'm any good. And it's all working. It doesn't matter. Buster matters. But it's hard not to notice that being pregnant is really working for me today, and I will soon be working for Seinfeld.

When we pull out of the parking lot after wrapping for the day, I say something to the Mister I've never said before: "They have to hire me. No one is going to be better than that."

Buster has not only gotten me a job, he has gotten me a job on what is sure to be a hugely high-profile and groundbreaking show.

My agent calls. Good news and bad news, she says.

Good news, they loved my piece, say the footage is cutting together great and they are sure Jerry will love it, too. Bad news, the crew told the producers I was one centimeter dilated and they feel it's just too much of a liability to have me in-studio the next day. The second part of the screen test is canceled. The producer says she feels terrible, because she is also a mom, but they just can't risk it.

This is totally fair, and I really should have kept my mouth closed about my birth canal opening, but I was just so tickled.

So, let's see. First, Buster gets me in the door by making me relax and not care if I'm any good; then he (okay, and my opening my mouth about my opening cervix) buys me a one-way ticket back to my hometown of Obscurity.

I'm disappointed, because it would have made a great story and because I do need to get a job, but I'm also relieved. There's a time for hustling and this obviously isn't it. No more clipping in my hair extensions and shoving my feet into presentable shoes and trying to impress. And to be totally honest, it feels like a reprieve, because it means I get to avoid performing again—especially for one of the most successful men in the history of television. Phew. I don't have to worry about the audition tomorrow. There is no longer anything on the horizon but getting the baby out safely.

I'll just put this Seinfeld thing on Buster's tab and perhaps consider that the baby is mocking the title of this book. Still, I intend to continue using him for a little "Serenity Now," to take his existence as my cue to accept that this latest career setback isn't a big deal in the big picture, the one in which Buster is now starring. Taking on this outlook is surprisingly effortless, not because I've become a better, more selfless and more grounded person, but because I've organically pulled some sort of George Costanza—in some ways, I'm kind of the opposite of who I used to be, going against all of my former instincts and habits. Buster Frank Breech is turned around and so am I, *yada, yada, yada.*

twenty-three

An Even Worse C-Word

It's the morning of my scheduled C-section, and I'm watching my dad and husband eat breakfast. I'm starving, but you aren't supposed to eat anything before surgery, so I sneak one bite of my dad's banana and gnaw the corner off my husband's bagel. I also may have chewed the end off a protein bar, but other than that, I didn't eat a thing or even drink water.

We drive to the hospital in Glendale in silence, after having taken a few snapshots on our front stairs. On the way home, four days from now, we will be parents.

The night before, my dad arrived from Northern California and we all went to the latest Michael Moore movie, *Capitalism: A Love Story*. I'm sure it was deeply stirring and educational, but it's hard to focus on the flawed nature of derivatives and ballooning mortgage payments when you are hours away from being sliced open. Eating my tub of popcorn, I couldn't help thinking about how vaginal birth is a much more compelling metaphor than a Cesarean, even when it comes to movie titles: *A Star Is Cut Out* or *C-Section of a Nation* or even *Unnaturally Born Killers* just doesn't sound right. I don't know how exactly Vietnam veteran Ron Kovic came out of his mother's womb, but the movie about his life is not called *Sliced Out on the Fourth of July*. Bruce Springsteen doesn't sing about being "Surgically Removed to Run," and "Removed with a Scalpel to be Wild" doesn't quite capture that rock-and-roll spirit.

Still, I'm sitting pretty, or as pretty as I can be having gained fifty-five pounds during my pregnancy, because earlier in the day I had my hair blown out and false eyelashes glued on. I won't be all glistening with sweat like the girls who get to wear the Vag of Honor, but at least I'll look my best in the first photos with baby. I'll look my best, or like a fat-ass drag queen, but either way, a scheduled C-section does allow one to enter motherhood with decent hair and a fresh pedicure.

We check into the hospital, and it's now two hours until surgery. I'm given a hospital gown, hooked up to a monitor to track the fetal heartbeat, stuck with an IV line for later and interviewed by a brusque intake nurse.

"When did you last eat?" she asks.

I look up at my dad, as if to ask him with my eyeballs, "Is this one of those times I'm supposed to lie?" but instead I let her know I took one bite of a banana.

"What? You ate a banana? I have to call the anesthesiologist. No eating before surgery. You were told that," she snaps. I decide this lady hates pregnant people, hates babies, hates life and surely has a thing against bananas.

"No, not a banana. A *bite* of a banana. I was nauseous, it was nothing, let's do this thing. Please," I beg the nurse.

There's a long, idiotic, dead-end discussion about whether I had a bite or bites, but she isn't budging and she tattles on me. They make me wait two more hours for the banana to digest, and a combination of the nerves and the hunger and the entire thirty-nine weeks of waiting for this moment only to have it pushed back by *two whole* hours has me on the verge of tears. Only the fear of dislodging my false eyelashes and my dad's measured tone keep me from tipping over the edge.

"Some rules are there for a reason," says my dad, softly. "It's for your own good. She's just doing her job. They don't want you to asphyxiate if something goes wrong and they have to put you under general. It's only two hours. Two hours is nothing." He pats my hair, which is sweet and strange, and so comforting I don't mind so much that he is mashing my do.

My dad is terrified to fly, and once he gets on an airplane, he gets very silent, drinks two glasses of wine in short order and goes glassy-eyed with a thin film of sweat on his upper lip. He looks like that now. Because he sees the baby's heart rate is normal, and because none of the medical professionals buzzing around seems worried about the baby, and because he is not filled with hormones and catastrophic ideas, and because he is not, as I am, insane, he isn't the least bit worried about the baby. He is worried about me. I am his baby. I'm thirty-nine years old, I have some crow's-feet and an IRA, but I am still his baby. I am to him what Buster is to me, a notion I've never fully understood until this moment.

"Dad, until you have kids, you don't understand anything about anything," I say, which is the kind of vague and meaningless statement that sounds deep when your glands are shooting an eight-ball of cortisol, adrenaline and endorphins into your system and you're high as hell on fight or flight.

The doula, Margie, arrives, in her faded jeans and embroidered shirt. It might seem strange to have a doula for a C-section, but, well, we already paid her and I like her and it can't hurt to have someone along who isn't a first-timer. We make small talk for two hours, and after one last ultrasound proving Buster is still Frank, it's time to wheel me into surgery.

Margie and my husband are asked to wait outside and get into some scrubs while I go into the operating room alone for my nerve block, so that I won't feel the lower half of my body when they cut into it. The anesthesiologist asks me to sit on the table sideways, with my feet dangling over the edge, and hunch over with my back out like a cat. He pokes around for a while, and says my "dura" (the membrane around my spinal cord) is tough and he can't quite get the needle in there.

Slouching over the table, I recall that in medical situations it's helpful to warn people that you might freak out. They take it pretty seriously.

"I don't want to alarm you, and I'll probably be fine, but there is a small chance I might freak out."

They are hesitant to give me any kind of anxiety-reducing drug, which could mess with the baby, and I am hesitant to ask for one, but I just need everyone to be on their toes in case I get the shakes or something. The forced cheerfulness in the room immediately increases by at least 27 percent as the team assures me I'm doing great. I'm not actually doing anything, just slouching and breathing, but I'll take any validation I can get. The doctor finally pokes through what I can only imagine is my fat dura and they lay me down and wait for the medicine to paralyze the lower half of my body. My arms are strapped down.

At this point, Margie and Daniel are allowed to come in and watch the show, though there is a big green medical sheet obscuring the business end of my body as they stand near my head. The medical team is chatting it up, they have some doctor friends in common, it's all very chipper, very ordinary, just another day at the office, another routine procedure, my body being sliced open to reveal a live baby for which I will be responsible the rest of my life, before and after which all manner of things could go wrong. I picture lots of rushing around, codes being called, the baby in an incubator, but the medical team is calm, doing their jobs, a carefully choreographed dance they've done hundreds of times.

If you know you are going to have a C-section and it's unavoidable, please think twice about reading the rest of this chapter. You will be fine, but maybe the less you know in advance the better.

As I start to lose feeling in my legs, it gets harder to breathe. The sensation in the lower half of my body—or lack thereof—is so disturbing, I keep asking where my legs are, as if being able to visualize their coordinates would make this less troubling. They give me an oxygen mask, but I still feel like I can't get air.

Margie assures me I'm not suffocating. "I'm looking right at the oxygen monitor. You're fine. The baby is fine."

It's hard to communicate through the oxygen mask, but I manage to inquire as to the location of my legs half a dozen more times.

I need distraction. There are way worse surgical situations than not being able to feel your lower half when you are totally awake. I know this. Still, it's so unbearable emotionally that it's unclear how long I can take it. This is hard to explain without sounding like someone who cuts her forearms and reads too much Plath, but I've never been afraid of dying. You leave the party and it's ashes to ashes and funk to funky. Being paralyzed, however, has always been my biggest fear. This paralysis isn't permanent, as it was for the aforementioned heroic vet Kovic, but the experience is beyond unpleasant.

Margie, seasoned birth professional that she is, warns me never to look up at the surgical light fixture, as the metal provides a reflective surface and I will be seeing the C. I avert my eyes and ask Margie to just describe the proceedings. She lets me know, right in my ear in her dulcet doula voice, that they have made the first cut. There might be the smell of burning flesh soon when the wound is cauterized, she explains. *Good to know.*

"Talk to me," I say to my husband, who is nothing if not laconic.

On our second date, I asked if I was talking too much and he begged me never to stop yammering. We made a deal that I would talk 85 percent of the time and he would fill in the rest for the duration of our relationship. He doesn't like to talk about himself and just isn't a loquacious guy. Now, he's blinking too much, looking a bit faint and mumbling, "Um, what should I talk about?"

I feel so bad. It's like asking a kitten to tap dance.

The doula delivers. I mean, she doesn't actually have to deliver, just deliver on her promise to make things easier, which she does by filling in the conversational gap, telling me how the incision looks, how the baby is doing, what to expect next. That was the best $1,500 we ever spent and I feel guilty that this is probably boring for her compared to a vaginal birth, but I'm grateful she's here. I wish there were doulas for everything difficult in life—job interviews, final exams, home buying, Thanksgiving with my family. I would like to grab Margie by the denim pant legs and never let her go. Looking into my husband's eyes, I love him for his quietness, because as much as I would enjoy a constant prattle, I know he's focused and present, and he's the kind of guy you want around during an emergency, emotional or otherwise. In the movies, when the woman is in labor, she curses the father for putting her in this position, and although I can't actually feel what position I'm in, I'm not cursing Daniel. I'm madly, painfully, achingly in love with him for the blinking and the terror and the forced preservation of a calm demeanor, because all of these things tell me how much we matter, Buster and me.

"Is it almost over? Where are my legs?" I ask again, still thinking knowing would make the paralysis more palatable. I tell myself it's just a few more minutes, that I'll get through it, that so many women have done this before me and I've never heard a single one talk about the creepy, helpless terror of a nerve block. What's that quote? *Whatever doesn't kill you just makes you wish you were dead.* No, it's supposed to make you stronger. Right. Right. This is making me stronger as I grit it out. It certainly beats the nerves firing at a time like this, and I should delight in the medical miracle of spinal blocks, but this is stretching the space-time continuum because I could swear my legs have been frozen for hours.

Small talk. Small talk. Small talk. Margie on the weather. The medical team continues to chat breezily like they do during surgeries on medical TV shows. Margie on whether we've chosen a baby name. Daniel blinking a lot. Margie reassuring me I'm getting enough oxygen. Daniel blinking and peering toward the sheet obscuring the procedure. Margie on how great this hospital is, because they let doulas in the operating room and because Adventist hospitals are known for their excellent food. Me on the leg thing again. Daniel finally grunting out the first syllable of a word, rest of word still unknown. Daniel looking longingly toward Margie when there is a brief silence. Margie reengaging small talk. Me willing to listen to any manner of conversation to forget that my skin, muscles, uterus are probably cleaved apart at this very moment, internal organs shifted aside, some set on top of my stomach for safekeeping to be returned after the baby is removed. The doctor's fingers are getting close to Buster. Frank No Name Buster. He is inside of my body and in minutes he will be out.

More blinking. Margie warning me the baby might not cry right away, so don't panic if we don't hear anything for a few seconds.

I don't know who it is, maybe a doctor, a nurse, the anesthesiologist, someone announces, "He's a chunky monkey," and I've never been more relieved than I am to hear the first fat joke about my son. I know no one would be joking if he didn't have all of his fingers and toes and appear to be in good working order. You don't start rhyming and referencing Ben & Jerry's flavors when things are going awry. Even someone with a spinal block, restraints and a nasty case of alarmism knows this on some visceral level.

After he's pronounced a chunky monkey, and the doctor says, "He was definitely breech . . . and definitely a boy" (I guess Buster presented with a big rump and typically swollen baby balls) I start bawling right there on the table, tears pooling around my oxygen mask. I'm trying not to choke on snot and shock and the weird mucus that collects when you're on your back and huge.

He is held up in the air like a bunch of grapes at a Sunday farmer's market, purple and shiny.

Until the second they bring him over to me and let me kiss his goopy red face, I am convinced that setting up a crib and buying a rug for his nursery and occasionally imagining he would be okay would all have cursed him, and that I would never, ever be lucky enough to get a real live healthy baby.

"Nine minutes," my husband says, because he's the kind of man who times things, and they hustle my husband over to cut the cord, calling him "Dad." Buster and Daniel leave so the medical team can weigh the baby and check his vitals while I get sewn up.

No matter how many tests told me otherwise and no matter how often I saw the graph of his heartbeat, even moments before they removed him and I could hear his heart thudding steady and strong on the fetal monitor, I was sure this was all a big mistake and that something would be wrong and everyone had missed it.

It takes half an hour to stitch the opening he left (I know this because my husband timed that, too) and I never stop sobbing with relief.

A nice Canadian nurse with Disney characters on her scrubs greets me in the recovery room. She hands me the baby to nurse him. He's all cleaned up, has a full head of light-colored hair, dimples on his cheeks. I know biology is supposed to make me think this way, but he really is beyond perfect. The Canadian woman helps me to nurse him for the first time, placing him on my chest, but it's easy.

Breast-feeding easily is the equivalent of having a big dick—no one will admit how good it feels, because it's really arbitrary and in no way means one is more of a man—but when that baby just takes to the boob, no pain, no trouble, I feel like I have a huge, swinging cock. I may have been so-so on nursing, and put off by all the wacky zealots who promote it, but I must admit, it gives me confidence. If nothing else, my baby, despite me, is doing something right. I'm feeding my baby, and all the nurses comment on his perfect latch and suddenly I want to pat myself on the back for taking that breast-feeding class and brag to anyone who will listen. *My baby is a chunky monkey and he has a perfect latch.*

We go to our room, with a huge window facing out toward the mountains, and the baby "rooms in." In other words, there is no nursery at our hospital. He's an hour old and he's ours full-time. I have a catheter, am on major opiates, can't walk, have been sliced open and still have an IV drip of fluids, but along with my husband I am now responsible for another person. We have no clue what we are doing.

Nurses, like angels, bring me a special juice cocktail they've invented: apple, prune, grapefruit, orange, all the juice flavors thrown together with ice and a straw.

Every sound Buster makes is adorable and terrifying. He sleeps all swaddled in a crisp hospital linen, white with red and blue trim. It's the "burrito" swaddle, a nurse tells us, as she places him in a bassinet across the room. Daniel is on a roll-away in the corner. I'm in a hospital bed, sedated and wired. And we're just sitting there with our baby.

Our baby.

twenty-four

Four Days in the Hole

I don't want to say hospitals play fast and loose with the pills after a C-section, but the bill from the pharmacy is over five grand. Next time I spend five grand on drugs, someone better throw in a hooker.

Again, if you know you are having a C-section, you may want to skip this chapter, because while some people have no trouble at all with the procedure, my recovery was gnarly.

There's no sleeping that first night.

For one thing, I'm staring at the bassinet, and back at my husband on a cot in the corner, and back at the baby, and I'm high on motherhood and narcotics and this is the best night of my life and I don't want to miss a thing (or ever sound like an Aerosmith song ever again).

Sure, I don't want to miss a thing, but being in the hospital after a C-section is not exactly conducive to rest anyway. The baby needs to nurse, my husband needs to change the kid's diapers because I can't move but Buster's bowels can, pediatricians need to check on the little guy, and it seems like every hour or so a nurse or a doctor needs to invade our room, clanging around almost cartoonishly like someone "accidentally" on purpose waking up a hungover teenager who's been sleeping twelve hours and should really be mowing the lawn.

Everyone has a job to do, which I understand, but it seems that job involves covering the hospital's ass so it doesn't get sued for not monitoring our vitals every four seconds.

They check my blood pressure constantly, which is painful because my upper arms are so swollen that the cuff squeezes the life out of me, causing my eyes to water until my dad begs them to use the old-school, crank-style BP machine. About every other time, they grudgingly succumb to my dad's pleas, but my arm is red and bruised nonetheless.

There's just overall a lot of barging. They barge in to take the baby's temperature, to make sure my catheter is still taped to my leg, to wash my privates, which to my surprise bleed profusely even after a C-section. I'm wearing giant maxipad things the likes of which you've never seen and the sponge baths they give my lady parts are dehumanizing for everyone involved.

Baby and Mom need lots of tests, no question, but somehow the way the disruptions are spaced makes me feel like a sleep experiment subject who eventually becomes psychotic. *What happens if we wait until the subject hits REM and just wake her up every single time and see if she can solve a simple math problem? Let's choose the perfect wake-up intervals to make sure her brain becomes scrambled and disorganized and her already fragile emotional state unravels and see how that goes.* I don't want to say the protocol is like torture, but I'm pretty sure John Yoo signed off on it.

To illustrate how many medications I'm given around the clock, I will just tell you that not only was the pharmacy bill five grand, the itemized list of drugs we later request is four pages long, single-spaced.

They give me pain pills, stool softeners, injections for nausea, suppositories for the constipation caused by the pain pills, pills for the itching caused by the morphine, gas tablets, Motrin and more.

My ankles and hands continue to swell up like a corpse floating in the Hudson.

There's a sudden piercing pain in my shoulder, like my clavicle is snapping, which convinces me I'm having some sort of heart attack. Since getting out of surgery, I have had pulsating pneumatic compression devices strapped to both my calves for the prevention of deep vein thrombosis, but perhaps they didn't work (other than the excellent job they do making me itchy and irritated). Now, I'm sure the gripping, gnawing feeling in my shoulder is a heart attack, a blood clot, or the beginnings of a stroke. The nurse tells me not to worry, that it is just gas. *Gas in my shoulder?* That is some bad, bad gas. They encourage me to get out of bed with my IV and walk the ward to shake the gas free. It takes half an hour to go ten yards, my husband pushing the baby along in the bassinet, but anything to get rid of this damn shoulder gas.

After the stroll, I hand Buster over to my dad. He is holding the baby in his lap, the 49ers game is on in the background, the baby yawns, and the sunlight from the window is landing on the baby's hair as he dozes in his grandfather's lap.

Listen, I don't want to miss a thing, but I'm kind of missing a lot of things.

Normally, I love opiates like Aerosmith loves . . . well, opiates, but I want to remember the way the sun looks reflecting on my dad's thick eyeglasses as he bounces my son and hums. I want to be less high. *What am I, high?*

I ask for weaker and fewer pain meds.

Days go by in a blur of pills and burst-open doors and baby checks and blood pressure readings and trapped gas bubbles until a headache hits like a stiletto to the side of my head. The nurse says this happens sometimes when the spinal cord gets nicked during a nerve block; no problem, they just open you up and patch it.

That's when, despite not having moved my bowels for days, I lose my proverbial shit. Before I even entered the hospital, I was sleep-deprived, and since then I have slept twenty minutes in thirty-six hours. I haven't pooped, I'm peeing into a bag, I can't even lift my own baby, my stomach is numb except where it burns, and now I might have to go back into surgery?

The heaving cries start, a few nurses materialize, offer to get a social worker, discuss giving me Xanax (yay!), which is contraindicated for breast-feeding (boo!) and I start having what feels like a bout of PTSD, flashbacks of losing feeling in my legs, of being sliced open, of the struggling for air, of the big old nothing that is supposed to be so routine. Can't go back. Can't.

"If you don't have this meltdown, I'll rub your feet," says my husband, in the same tone he now uses with Buster. So I stop and he rubs. Suicide hotlines should consider this tactic.

"You're just tired," he adds, massaging, and the nurses take pity on us and offer to babysit for a couple of hours, wheeling the baby in his bassinet out to the nursing station.

There's a chance the headache is actually a withdrawal symptom from not stepping gradually down off the dolls. The prescription? A large cup of medical-grade coffee that probably costs my insurance company $97, and it works. In your face, Starbucks, you ain't the most expensive cup of coffee in town. One cure for a symptom caused by another cure.

Between the C-section and the chasing my own tail by treating ills caused by pills treating other ills, I feel this experience turning me against my sweet, sweet drugs and Western medicine in general (which seems unfair, being that a breech baby would likely have ripped me apart without the surgical intervention in the first place. I should consider myself lucky to be enjoying the age of modern obstetrics).

Ironically, after the coffee I sleep, with the baby under the care of a nursing assistant named Delilah, who I'm pretty sure is breaking a rule but is mending my psyche.

After a while, she brings the baby in to nurse. The breast-feeding is constant. At one point I think the baby has peed on me, but the rush of liquid is really just my milk coming in (as opposed to colostrum, the low-volume nutrient moms make first) and spilling out, gushing down my hospital gown. My boobs are engorged, a solid D cup if not bigger now, and hard as bone.

The baby has a little jaundice, nothing serious, but this means more barging and checking.

Buster gets a hearing test, during which he's hooked up to a computer while wearing little headphones. He is so cute with his headphones, and my husband takes pictures of the whole procedure, including a shot of the computer screen that reads "Pass."

Every day, a lady comes in wanting the boy's name for his birth certificate. We got nothing. Everyone said we'd know when we saw him, but all we know is that he is not an Edward, a James, a Finn, a Mickey or a Shane.

My dad keeps us company, blathering on about everything from holes in the 49ers' defense to his new part-time job tutoring kids, and the various challenging students he is attempting to teach math. He's going on and on and my husband does something he never does. He cuts off someone who is speaking.

"What did you say that kid's name was?"

"Huh?" says my dad. "Oh. Nathaniel. Anyway, Nathaniel was

upset that he couldn't figure out his times tables, so what I did was I—"

"That's it. Nathaniel. Nathaniel James. That's the name," announces my husband.

Yes.

It's not too common and it's not too weird. And it suits him. Little Nathaniel.

We arrived as two people with a Frank Breech fetus called Buster and we are leaving as the parents of a boy named Nathaniel James, born seven pounds, seven ounces.

Despite the strain of constant tests and medications, we have fallen in love with our nursing staff. They help the baby latch, they know how to swaddle, they reassure us when he makes a funny sound, and they burp him with ease and confidence. We are terrified to leave and don't feel ready, and we stay there until literally the last minute of our allotted four days has passed. We put the baby in his best outfit, a gift from my girlfriend Lynette, tiny white pants and a blue-and-white-striped kimono top with matching hat. We pack up the bag of time-fillers we thought we would need, a bag that was never even unzipped, filled with a deck of cards, a game of Boggle and a stack of brand-new books. They wheel me out toward the front door.

Legally, they have to wheel you out, but in my case, it's not just for show. I'm still not walking very well. My husband leaves me with the baby while he pulls the car around and I'm alone with Nathaniel for the first time. There's a four-day-old baby in a hat in my lap.

We get him into his car seat and I sit in the backseat beside him, holding up his tiny noggin as we drive home. With every bump in the road, my tender insides are screaming, and so is the baby.

Daniel is driving with the approximate speed and deliberateness of a stoner passing a police station, and my Gandhi of a husband has greeted fatherhood with a strange bout of road rage. "What are you doing, motherfucker? I need you to *move the fuck out of my lane.*" He's in charge of our family now, the only one with full faculties, and Daddy has to get us the fuck home.

twenty-five

Day One: The Infinite Pint

It's my first day out of the hospital and I'm feeling pretty wrecked. Haven't even had a chance to check out my new slice, but I have run my fingers over it and I will tell you, they need a little extra room to remove the frank breech types. Seems about five inches or so. I'm okay with the scar in principle; I just don't want to see it yet.

My husband frantically runs out to the store and comes back with $700 worth of groceries, which must be his form of nesting, like when I was nine months pregnant and decided to order twenty-four Magic Erasers and remove every mark on every wall in our house. We don't just have everything. We have three of everything: three jugs of prune juice (it's been five days since I've gone number two), three boxes of every Lean Cuisine I like, three bottles of three different kinds of gas drops for babies, three tubs of pasta salad from the deli counter.

Despite having birthed a baby and a placenta, I still appear almost as pregnant as when I went in for surgery, which I wasn't expecting. I had deluded myself into thinking that despite my above-average weight gain, I would waltz out of the hospital not totally back to normal, but at least in my chubby jeans. No. I look virtually the same, except maternity clothes look terrible now, because they are designed to highlight the bump, which is exactly what you don't want unless you like people asking you when you're due and having to lie and say, "Next month. So excited." My legs are still so bulky that my ankles and knees are hard to differentiate from the overall fluff of leg flesh. My wrists are sore, so I wear one of those carpal tunnel splints on both hands. My new giant shoes don't even fit, so it's slippers full-time. When the baby takes a nap, I sit in bed with my laptop and order some men's dress shirts from Target because the old clothes aren't even close to fitting and the pregnancy clothes all feature a new mom's worst enemy: empire waists.

Because of the baby's jaundice, I nurse him every two hours or more. In between, we take him out for a little sunshine in ten-minute increments as prescribed by the hospital pediatrician, and then it's back to more nursing. Nurse, burp, diaper, sunshine, rinse, repeat.

Sometimes it's kind of nice to find yourself living a cliché. Deliriously happy and deliriously tired mom, that's me. Mom. I'm someone's mom. He is my son.

You know the surreal sensation that accompanies being pregnant, what I always think of as a Talking Heads moment ("You may find yourself in a beautiful house, with a beautiful wife. You may ask yourself, well, how did I get here?")? It's magnified a hundred times when one day there is no baby, and the next, there is your baby. At times I think to myself, "Surely, this isn't real. This has been fun, but I wonder when Nate's parents are coming to pick him up." I don't mean this in a detached way, as in, I better get on Prozac because I don't love my baby or feel connected to him, but the opposite, something more like winning the lottery but still buying generic catsup the next day because it hasn't sunk in that you're loaded.

For someone who wasn't baby crazy, who didn't really get babies at all, who never actually held a baby until I was four months pregnant and snuggled Cassandra's baby for a minute or two, I do all the disgustingly mommyish things actual moms do, like smell his head and take pictures of him incessantly and become convinced that I'm not biased at all but that my baby actually is extra adorable with fantastic hair and an exceptional disposition, which he surely inherited from his dad.

The sensations I'm having now, the baby "high" and the rubbing his velvety arms and the crying because I can't poop or sleep and the sad-sack thoughts when I catch my bloated reflection and the dreamlike smacking myself over being his mom and him not being in my stomach anymore but instead sitting there in his bouncy seat, I know this has all been said and done and felt before. Maybe by you. But instead of that taking away from its value, somehow, today, it seems to add to it. Instead of scoffing at the human experience, I'm just giving in.

I remember when we were walking along the beach in Avila trying to decide whether to have a baby and thinking there aren't that many main courses on the menu of life. Despite wanting to be terminally unique, at some point you just have to order the chicken or the steak. Maybe the surf and turf. Because there are only so many entrées at the cosmic table. And here I am with my baby, like a billion and a half mothers before me, and we all want to hear that our children are chunky monkeys, and that we are not, and that's where I find magic where I least expected it, right in the schmaltziness.

It feels so good to have what the rest of you are having. I'm happy I'm actually welcome at the table, even if I don't quite have a grasp of the table manners yet. I earned my seat not by being special but just by being deliciously ordinary. All I really have to do is eat what's in front of me, a bite at a time. All I really have to do to be a good mom is love this creature, which I do despite my fears that I couldn't.

The feelings are so sweet that maybe I've skipped right to dessert. There aren't many offerings here, either, and that's the best part of motherhood so far, that we're all telling the same stories and delving our cold spoon into one infinite pint of baby bliss.

twenty-six

My Mother, the Rabbi and
a Bag of Crap

B uster is one month old today.

And I think I am finally ready to tell the story about the rabbi, my estranged mother and a bag of shit, and how this only partially holy trinity converged at my home one Tuesday afternoon.

When Buster was eight days old, we invited a rabbi over to circumcise the kid. My husband—not a Jew—was okay with the snip-snip but thought it was creepy to turn the whole situation into a party. Fair enough. So it was going to be just the two of us, until he started suggesting it might be nice to have my mom there, my mom who I haven't talked to in over a year now.

Just before the baby was born, a package arrived addressed to the unborn child from "Grandma Strasser." Inside were a hand-knit orange stuffed dinosaur, a tiny sweater with pockets and a hood, and a powder blue blanket. Though she hadn't called me since my brother told her I was pregnant, it looked as though she had been knitting ever since.

There was a note to the baby that simply said, "Grandma can't wait to meet you."

I cried my fucking eyes out with that orange dinosaur in my hand because I was hormonal, and it was a week before my baby was due, and my mother was reaching out in her own stilted way, and while it would be nice if she could say "sorry" or "I miss you," I stood on my stoop fully aware that some people speak with yarn.

That woman let me down in such a profound way that just the sound of her clearing her throat too loudly makes me want to toss her purse out of a moving car. Try as I may, I haven't been able to process the backlog of anger at her even after all these years, which has made me an impatient, puerile, irrational daughter. Yes, the woman put me on many a Greyhound bus when I was in elementary school, but I don't know how to stop making her pay, so I just stop talking to her.

It's kind of a mom sabbatical. I take one every few years or so.

Somehow, between the knit creature's baleful look and the post C-section narcotics, my husband convinces me that we should invite my mom to the *bris*.

Also, when we went to the rabbi's Web site, there was a checklist of things we needed for the procedure—gauze pads, kosher wine, ointment and other items the acquisition of which was impossible as I could still barely get up and down and my husband couldn't leave me alone with the baby. I was a mommy and I needed a mommy. I really needed my mommy.

My husband calls her for me, and as he predicted, she accepts the invite on very short notice, offering to pick up everything we need plus a platter of bagels and lox. I can hear her voice over the phone, and the tone suggests something like enthusiasm, maybe even exuberance. It heartens me that my chronically depressed mom would not only sound elated to hear from us but would also drive five hours from Vegas to see her new grandson at the drop of a yarmulke, salve in hand.

So, with the rabbi and my mother heading our way for the afternoon ceremony, my bowels, which as you already know have been stopped up, finally decide to work after more than a week.

The resulting poop clogs the decrepit toilet in our old house.

At this point, I can't bend, lift or twist. So, I sit there on the potty with my head in my hands just trying to think my way out of this mess. The rabbi and my mother are converging on the place in half an hour, my week-old son is stirring in the next room with his dad, and I am hovering over—and up—Shit's Creek.

I am not now nor have I ever been one of those women who impresses guys by being really open and carefree about their gas and bodily functions. Even writing this makes me vaguely uncomfortable. Sometimes I wish I was that fart-in-your-face girl (I honestly hate even typing the word F-A-R-T), but there came a point in my twenties when I realized two things: I don't dance, and I don't enjoy talking about gas or bowel movements. When I embraced being fundamentally inhibited, it changed my life. I am not the girl pretending to think gas is funny or grimacing my way through the conga line at a wedding.

While I have few, if any, emotional boundaries, I make up for it by being private, almost proper, about the physical realm. I would like the world to believe that I don't poop but instead excrete waste through my skin, like a frog. Never have I indicated in any way to the Mister, up until this moment, that anything noxious ever comes out of my ass, but now I'm screwed.

"Baby," I yell, sheepishly, "I have a problem." That's when my husband rushes to the bathroom door. I start sobbing because I'm freaked out and exhausted and I don't want this magical Jewish ritual to be marred by the smell of feces wafting through the house, *my* feces, and I certainly don't want my husband seeing, smelling or experiencing my waste in any way, but I'm out of options. I wash my hands like I can cleanse myself of this whole situation.

He hands me the baby and runs to the garage for some sort of drain snake. I try to place my thoughts elsewhere, so that I can easily delete this memory in the future. I bounce the boy and look out the window at Koreatown.

There is some running back and forth from the garage to the front door, to the bathroom in back. I hear him call the plumber, who can't make it until tomorrow. He calls the hardware store to see if they have a larger snake; they do not. I bounce the boy and watch the clock. Fifteen minutes to go.

It is at this moment that I glance outside the window again and see my husband running gingerly along the side of the house holding a plastic bag.

It takes my mind a moment to process (again, drugs, lack of sleep, major surgery, sudden life-changing transition to motherhood, heavy emotional family issues about to be addressed, impending removal of my baby's foreskin).

There it is. My husband walk-running around the side of the house carrying—as one might a goldfish won at a county fair—a bag of toilet water and the offending, drain-clogging crap that he has somehow liberated from the bowl.

Nothing says your life has crossed over like seeing your husband carry a bag of your shit.

If one could die of cringing, I would.

This is all my fault, I tell myself, for not better orchestrating my life, for having a breech baby and a C-section, for moving to this old house just weeks before the baby's birth because I couldn't make up my mind any sooner, for all the chaos of unpacked boxes and curtains not hung. I want everything to be slender and clean and tucked away and predictable, but I can't go back and I smell Buster's fuzzy head just to get a hit of the good stuff.

This, too, shall pass, I tell myself, just as that poop did through my colon.

Until now, I didn't even discuss going number one with my husband and now I'm anxiously running to the front door to find out how it went when he hand-delivered a bag of number two to the trash can out front.

"No problem," he says, trying to pass it off. "All fixed."

A tacit agreement that this didn't happen is made.

Before the rabbi arrives—a bearded man right out of Central Casting—my mom shows up. She has been driving for hours, so her lime green linen shirt is a bit rumpled, but I can tell she has dressed up. She is carrying a lavish platter of bagels, cream cheese and lox for fifteen, as well as a bag with doubles and triples of all the items on the rabbi's list. When she opens the door, I hug her and point to the baby, sleeping in his bouncy seat perched on the sofa. She strains to keep a neutral expression on her face, but tears are landing on her shirt. She doesn't make a move to wipe them away, because her face is still trying to say, "This is no big deal." I hand her the baby and she cries right onto his blankie, which she must recognize from her months of knitting it.

"He's beautiful," she says. And she manages to sound a way she never has before. *Maternal.*

And just like that, we commence making small talk about Buster, his dimples, will his eye color change, does he know what terrible thing is about to happen to his pee-pee. We have a nosh. Like the unspoken agreement never to discuss the contents of the bag, my mother and I silently conspire to act as though the past year, and many of the years before that, have not been crap.

The rabbi arrives, and dips a cloth into some wine while gathering the four of us to talk about the "covenant" and the idea that a circumcision happens on the baby's eighth day because there is no eighth day of the week and so the concept is to transcend the earthly plain. Or something like that. I don't know. Anything a guy with a long beard who has done fifteen thousand snips has to say seems deep. And we give the child a Hebrew name—David—because my stepfather's last name was Davidson and I know this will make my mom happy. When my stepfather was around, I could deal with my mother. He was a buffer, like the baby will be.

At the rabbi's request, my mom holds the baby and lets him suck on the wine-soaked corner of a cloth. This is anesthesia, old school and Old Testament style. The baby is sucking on that Manischewitz-soaked rag like maybe his gentile half is taking over, which gives us an easy laugh.

After looking around, the rabbi sets up shop on my desk, because that's where the sunlight filters in and he wants a clear view. My husband holds the cloth in the baby's mouth as the rabbi does his thing. Thirty seconds later, with barely a peep from the boy, it's all over.

Before leaving, the rabbi gives us instructions on how and when to apply the ointment and tells us to bury the foreskin in the dirt to show God we are earthy. It feels like I've been sucking on a wine cloth of my own, but I'm just tipsy with a double shot of relief and gratitude; my husband not only fixed the toilet, but he duct-taped over the mom problem, which can never be truly repaired but can at least be patched and repatched. Now she isn't just my mother but my son's grandmother, and I would be an asshole to rob my son of his grandma because I can't forgive her.

The rabbi is a man gifted with babies.

He tells us to stay calm, always calm, so your baby will do the same. This isn't always easy for me, because I love that little fucker so much that the idea of making a mistake, of not knowing what he needs or failing him, the worry that something may be broken in his body or mind that I can't fix, the idea that I don't have the patience or sweetness or wisdom to deserve him, well, that is the big bag of shit my soul carries around.

The rabbi leaves. My mom heads back to Vegas, careful not to overstay her welcome. Later that night, as we're eating leftover bagels and cream cheese, I send my mother a photo my husband took of her holding Buster, tears dotting her green shirt, mouth slightly turned down at the corners, staring down at her first grandchild. She e-mails back, "Please keep the pictures coming, love Grandma." And we bury the foreskin in the front yard.

twenty-seven

I Said a Lot of Things

I was full of pronouncements before I had this baby.

Forget those new moms who whine incessantly about not having time to shower; in a triumph of will and excellent planning, I was going to be the impeccably groomed mother of a newborn. I would make time for blowouts and basic hygiene, because I'm vain, own seventeen tubes of lip gloss, and refuse to wear too-tight Juicy Couture sweatpants and be all sacrifice-y and blah.

Cut to me sitting around in my own filth with breast milk stains on my XL men's shirt from Target, spit-up on my maternity jeans and hair so dirty that when I finally go to the salon, the hairdresser asks me, with more genuine curiosity than disdain, "How long has it been since you washed your hair?"

"Maybe three days?" I lie, before playing the new mom card.

And there I am, flying right in the puffy face of my own naïve declarations. On top of which, I have to ask the hairdresser to hurry it up—the sitter is waiting. *The sitter is waiting.* This is my life now. It's not unusual for me to take a hooker shower in front of the bathroom sink with a couple of baby wipes and almost no shame. I'm this person.

Like I said, I made a lot of pronouncements.

I proclaimed I would never be one of those moms who has entire conversations about my child's poop. Yet last night I Googled "green poop" on my iPhone while nursing and have now had lengthy conversations with several moms about the causes and potential dangers of green poop. (Just so you know, poop is only concerning if it's white, black or red, according to Babycenter.com.) Now I get it, I get the poop talk. As a new mom, I'm just trying to do right by Buster and he is very limited in his modes of communication so he has to let his poop do the talking. We have even photographed the green poop, lest our idea of green and our pediatrician's differ. Mint green? Forest green? Mossy green? Let's break out our camera and show you the exact hue. This is my life now. On my camera, *there is more than one picture of my child's poop.* I'm this person.

There was a time I loathed homes that were filled with baby accoutrements. Now there is no Mozart-playing swing center or Velcro-enhanced baby swaddle I won't buy. Whereas I used to think the baby industry was out to get me, I'm now out to get any crutch that will help me entertain my baby. The house looks like a Chuck E. Cheese's after an earthquake.

To anyone who would listen, I announced that you would never catch me in any kind of Mommy and Me bullshit, or one of these new mom support groups. Now I'm desperate to fit one into my schedule. If you have been a mother for even one day longer than I have, you know things I don't and you can help me.

Whereas I used to assume I would never fit in with women who would populate these classes, that I would never be one of the bland, stroller-lugging mom masses who gives a green crap about the superiority of Desitin or organic muslin burp cloths, now I practically molest moms I see on the street, at restaurants, anywhere, peppering them with questions: Do you like that baby carrier? Does it hurt your back? How long did you breast-feed? Did your baby ever get a rash on her cheeks? What pediatrician do you go to? How long does your baby sleep? When did she start sleeping through the night? What exactly is a Sleep Sheep?

I take feverish notes, especially about whatever DVD or book she says was the magical sleep maker. I buy it all.

When I get a mom in my clutches who seems to know what she's doing, something I deduce from the effortless way she snaps a car seat into a stroller frame or wipes the drool from her child's chin with a bumble-bee-covered burp cloth that materializes from somewhere on her person, I don't stop at the easy questions; I pry her for information about vaccines, eating solid foods, how soon after the baby she and her husband had sex and anything else she seems open enough to reveal. I always ask her how long it took to lose the baby weight, but I can tell already that even though I'm still big, my eating has gone back to normal, and soon my size will, too.

Just like the new kid in school who is trying to fit in, I'm starting to inch up to the mom crowd, to figure out what they wear and how they act and think. The clerk at the store where I took my breast-feeding workshop tells me that the Monday afternoon support group is empty, because all the moms go to the Mommy and Me movie at the mall that day. Get here early on Tuesdays, she adds, because it's standing room only. And I realize the moms travel in a flock, and maybe I'd be better off getting in formation than flying solo. If I go where they go, maybe I can learn what they know. Part of me is still wary of joining, because I want to do everything my own way, but I'm starting to think my own way sucks and that there is an inherent wisdom to the flock. Besides, in every social situation I've ever been in, I always find the one other girl who feels like a complete outsider and we become friends, even if that bond is at least in part based on judging everyone else who seems happier and better adjusted.

What I'm saying is this: Yes, I am sitting here in public (very public, at the public library, in fact, where a girl can look a mess and stink a little without bothering any of the homeless men checking their e-mail and reading *USA Today*) wearing what is really kind of a nightgown with ankle socks and sneakers. This is my life now. I don't care. I'd rather not run into any ex-boyfriends, but I don't really care.

I said a lot of things before. I have the one stretch mark, but I don't mind it.

I said I would never use a picture of my child as my profile photo anywhere, because I would rather lose my identity in more subtle ways. Already my cell phone wallpaper is a photo of Buster in a blue knit cap, no me, no dad, just the boy. That is a gateway baby photo, which can only lead to more serious use of the baby's picture to stand in for my own. It's happening.

I said only stone-cold bores and anti-intellectual twats spoke for their infants, imbuing them with all kinds of adult thoughts and feelings they could never, ever possess, the way a spinster announces that Mr. Fluffy loves *Friday Night Lights* but doesn't care for the sound of the mailman's voice. That was before my soul got splashed by maternal hormones and dried off only to find it appropriate to say, "Buster is flirting with you" or "Buster loves Jimmy Page guitar solos" or "Buster can't wait to see Grandpa" or "Buster feels so dapper in his cardigan" or "Buster just loves his bath." Like I know what the fuck that guy thinks or feels.

The fact is: I don't know shit. I literally don't know shit about shit. I don't know why his poop is sometimes green or if it matters, I don't know what goes on in my child's mind, if anything, or how best to plan his nap and feeding schedule so he sleeps through the night, or when to stop swaddling him or what causes a baby rash or if I should really stop eating milk or nuts or soy or whether he really needs a hepatitis B vaccine or if he's fussier than other babies or cries more or sleeps less or if, in fact, he is totally average.

It's like I met a guy, fell in love at first sight, flew to Vegas to get married that day, and woke up to find I was madly in love with this man but didn't know what he took in his coffee. I don't know Buster, or if there is much to know yet. Sometimes I don't know why he cries, or what exactly he needs, or if he has eaten too much or not enough. I just know I love him, because when I listen to John Denver songs and look down at him I cry right onto his now bald head with a feeling of categorical euphoria (Jesus, could I possibly have the "postpartum elation" I so mocked Nancy O'Dell for possessing?). Later, I cry because my stomach still hurts from the C-section and I just want to put him down but he needs to be rocked all the livelong day.

Sure, I have become some of the people I wanted to punch, but I've softened, and now I don't really want to punch anyone. I do, however, want to give a light shove to a certain breed of mom who seems to get her sustenance from judging other moms. These staunch, disapproving types do a lot of preaching about how motherhood should be done. From Gerber to Ferber, they have strong, myopic opinions on all things baby-related and disdain for women who don't do what they do. Listen, I'm not interested in debating whether moms should work, or kids should cry it out, or families should cosleep. As much as I used to long for people to just tell me what to do, I don't think it serves us to be prescribing and finger-pointing. While I'm thirsty for information, I gag on the flavor of maternal contempt.

As the saying goes, it takes a village to raise a child, women all pitching in to care for the babies in the community; only now it's a digital village, a world in which we all read the same Web sites and articles and blogs. Parenthood is hard enough without message boards and experts in our "village" telling us that pacifiers are evil, or working moms are selfish, or feeding your baby on a three-hour schedule is the only way to ensure he doesn't become a spoiled monster. Back in the day, mothers didn't sit around chirping about how their way was best; they just shut up and put your baby in their sling so you could go gather yams for dinner. Let's not be bound by our scrutiny, but by our communal attempt not to screw up.

I realize I'm preaching about not being preachy, and I sense already that I will have to keep this in check.

I will try never to judge what you do, though I will want to know all about it. "Whatever gets you through the night" is not just the chorus of my new favorite lullaby; it is also my mom mantra.

There are parenting theories and philosophies that bombard you at every stage of your child's life. Every milestone means collecting and synthesizing more data. Deciphering the best way to do things, that's an intellectual exercise, and learning is generally something I'm good at and comfortable with—as opposed to being a loving mother to a new creature, which is terrifying and thrilling and sometimes frustrating and boring.

So I keep Googling and grilling, but just when I have a handle on some small aspect of baby rearing, and I'm tempted to start bragging about finding the perfect sleep sack or bedtime routine, he goes and changes on me. He's a guitar that can't be tuned once and welded in place. In fact, it's starting to sink in that it's not a question of how well I tune him, but how well I stay in tune with him.

I'm hoping I can't go wrong if I just enjoy the kid without breaking him.

Buster smiles now. First, they were fake-out gas smiles, but now he seems to smile with his whole body. When that baby grins at me in the morning, squirming on his changing table, it's like a shot of morphine right to my heart. I spend the rest of the day chasing the dragon.

ACKNOWLEDGMENTS

I wasted a lot of time fantasizing about this section of the book while I was supposed to be actually writing the book, so it's already been written many times in my mind.

In no particular order, I want to thank both people and places. Thanks to the Los Feliz Branch Public Library, where much of this book was written. While some of you library ladies gave me the stink eye when I broke out my thermos of coffee and occasionally answered a call from the sitter, you were mostly welcoming and it was a haven for me.

My literary agent, Anthony Mattero, didn't just sell my book; he sold me on the idea that I could write it. I will forever be in his debt. Anthony, for being a young, unmarried dude and reading so much about vaginas and contractions, I adore you. Thanks to my editor at NAL, Tracy Bernstein, for being meticulous, thorough, thoughtful, patient, and most of all a successful working mother.

The writer Bill Simmons once told me, "Just keep your fingers moving." This is what chronic overthinkers need to hear. He may not remember saying it, but I won't forget hearing it. To my friend and colleague Ted Kamp, your confidence in me is baffling and boundless. You are never without an overflow of brilliant ideas and a combination of darkness and optimism that I've come to love. Your kids are so lucky.

To my once pregnant and now mom friends, thanks for letting me be part of your crew.

Adam Carolla, I could never say this to your face because both of us have impaired social skills, but I love you for giving me a chance. You hate everything, and you don't hate me, and that gave me the balls I needed. Without you, this book would not exist.

Thanks to Karen Wang-Lavelle, Lexi Strumor, Rob Eshman, Michele Ku, Frank Conniff, Danny Seckel, Gary Lucy, Marc S. Klein, Christy Lemire, Joel Stein, Ben Mankiewicz, Pamela Redmond Satran, Stephen Schwartz and Terrence McDonnell for their belief in me and support at various turning points in my career.

Last, my husband and both of my parents are heroes for helping watch the baby while I wrote. Mom, you take some serious shit in these pages, and while you may not have always been a great parent, you are a great sport. Dad, for being the sunniest person on the planet, you are my idol. To my husband and son, my only wish is to continue to deserve you. Even now, typing the word "son," I get teary.